Veterinary Guide to Animal Breeds

Veterinary Guide to Animal Breeds

Beth Vanhorn
Practice Manager, CVT
Banfield Pet Hospital
Lancaster, PA
Adult Education Instructor, Veterinary Assistant Program
Dauphin County Technical School
Harrisburg, PA

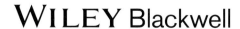

This edition first published 2018
© 2018 John Wiley & Sons

The right of Beth Vanhorn to be identified as the author of this work has been asserted in accordance with law.

Registered Offices
John Wiley & Sons, Inc., 111 River Street, Hoboken, NJ 07030, USA

Editorial Office
John Wiley & Sons, Inc. (111 River Street, Hoboken, New Jersey 07030)

For details of our global editorial offices, customer services, and more information about Wiley products visit us at www.wiley.com.

Wiley also publishes its books in a variety of electronic formats and by print-on-demand. Some content that appears in standard print versions of this book may not be available in other formats.

Library of Congress Cataloging-in-Publication Data

Names: Vanhorn, Beth, author.
Title: Veterinary guide to animal breeds / Beth Vanhorn.
Description: Hoboken, NJ : John Wiley & Sons, 2017. | Includes
    bibliographical references and index.
Identifiers: LCCN 2017003599 (print) | LCCN 2017010061 (ebook) |
    ISBN 9781119299721 (pbk.) | ISBN 9781119299745 (Adobe PDF) |
    ISBN 9781119299752 (ePub)
Subjects: LCSH: Animals–Identification. | Veterinary medicine–Handbooks, manuals, etc.
Classification: LCC SF745 .V36 2017 (print) | LCC SF745 (ebook) | DDC 636.089–dc23
LC record available at https://lccn.loc.gov/2017003599

Cover image: Courtesy of Beth Vanhorn
Cover design by Wiley

Set in 10/12pt WarnockPro by Aptara Inc., New Delhi, India

Printed and bound in Singapore by Markono Print Media Pte Ltd

10 9 8 7 6 5 4 3 2 1

Contents

Preface *ix*
About the Companion Website *ix*

1   Dog Breed Identification *1*
        Objectives *1*
1.1   Introduction *1*
1.2   Characteristics of Dogs *1*
1.3   Classes of Breeds *1*
1.4   Summary *4*

2   Cat Breed Identification *5*
        Objectives *5*
2.1   Introduction *5*
2.2   Characteristics of Cats *5*
2.3   Classes of Breeds *5*
2.4   Summary *8*

3   Rabbit Breed Identification *9*
        Objectives *9*
3.1   Introduction *9*
3.2   Characteristics of Rabbits *9*
3.3   Types of Rabbits *9*
3.4   Summary *11*

4   Guinea Pig Breed Identification *13*
        Objectives *13*
4.1   Introduction *13*
4.2   Characteristics of Guinea Pigs *13*
4.3   Types of Guinea Pigs *13*
4.4   Summary *14*

5   Pocket Pet Breed Identification *15*
        Objectives *15*
5.1   Introduction *15*
5.2   Characteristics of Mice *15*
5.3   Characteristics of Rats *15*
5.4   Characteristics of Hamsters *16*
5.5   Characteristics of Chinchillas *17*
5.6   Characteristics of Hedgehogs *17*
5.7   Characteristics of Gerbils *17*
5.8   Characteristics of Ferrets *18*
5.9   Summary *18*

6   **Avian Breed Identification**   *21*
        Objectives   *21*
6.1   Introduction   *21*
6.2   Characteristics of Companion Birds   *21*
6.3   Orders of Companion Birds   *22*
6.4   Summary   *24*

7   **Reptile Species Identification**   *25*
        Objectives   *25*
7.1   Introduction   *25*
7.2   Characteristics of Reptiles   *25*
7.3   Types of Reptiles   *26*
7.4   Summary   *27*

8   **Amphibian Species Identification**   *29*
        Objectives   *29*
8.1   Introduction   *29*
8.2   Characteristics of Amphibians   *29*
8.3   Types of Amphibians   *29*
8.4   Summary   *31*

9   **Cattle Breed Identification**   *33*
        Objectives   *33*
9.1   Introduction   *33*
9.2   Characteristics of Cattle   *33*
9.3   Types of Cattle   *34*
9.4   Summary   *35*

10   **Equine Breed Identification**   *37*
        Objectives   *37*
10.1   Introduction   *37*
10.2   Characteristics of Equines   *37*
10.3   Types of Equines   *38*
10.4   Summary   *40*

11   **Swine Breed Identification**   *41*
        Objectives   *41*
11.1   Introduction   *41*
11.2   Characteristics of Swine   *41*
11.3   Types of Swine   *41*
11.4   Breeds of Swine   *42*
11.5   Summary   *45*

12   **Sheep Breed Identification**   *47*
        Objectives   *47*
12.1   Introduction   *47*
12.2   Characteristics of Sheep   *47*
12.3   Classes of Sheep   *47*
12.4   Breeds of Sheep   *49*
12.5   Summary   *52*

13   **Goat Breed Identification**   *53*
        Objectives   *53*
13.1   Introduction   *53*

13.2   Characteristics of Goats   *53*
13.3   Classes of Goats   *53*
13.4   Breeds of Goats   *54*
13.5   Summary   *56*

14   Poultry Breed Identification   *57*
         Objectives   *57*
14.1   Introduction   *57*
14.2   Characteristics of Poultry   *57*
14.3   Classes of Poultry   *57*
14.4   Breeds of Poultry   *60*
14.5   Summary   *67*

15   Alternative Production Animal Breed Identification   *69*
         Objectives   *69*
15.1   Introduction   *69*
15.2   Alternative Animal Production Systems   *69*
15.3   Common Alternative Production Animal Species   *69*
15.4   Summary   *76*

Appendix   *77*
Index   *107*

Preface

Animal breed identification is vital to many careers and production industries. A comprehensive understanding of domesticated animal species and breeds is important for those working in or wishing to seek a career in veterinary fields, animal agriculture, and pet-related industries, and for the general public, as this resource will provide valuable information in the field of animal production and animal science. The purpose of this book is to provide a comprehensive list of domesticated animals, both large and small, to allow the reader to develop skills in species and breed identification. It consists of 15 chapters that recognize large, small exotic, and production animal species that have been domesticated or raised in a human environment for use in the animal industry. Each chapter discusses the species characteristics and provides identi-

fication information on breeds, classes, or types of each animal species. The book also provides supplementary information, with animal breed lists for each chapter and Power Point slides for ease of learning how to identify each animal, together with review questions at the end of each chapter. The author believes that the basic layout of the text offers professionals and students alike a useful tool under one cover to learn how to identify domesticated animal species and breeds. This approach provides a learning experience to preview animal species within the veterinary and animal science industries and presents an area to which current professionals can turn in order to identify unknown or unrecognizable animals that may be encountered in the animal profession.

About the Companion Website

This book is accompanied by a companion website:

www.wiley.com/go/vanhorn/breeds

The website includes:

- Multiple choice questions
- Breed identification worksheets
- Teaching PowerPoints

1

Dog Breed Identification

1.1 Introduction

Dogs are direct descendants of the wolf. The wolf is classified as *Canis lupus* and the dog as *Canis familiaris*. Dogs have become the second most popular animal in pet ownership, with over 73 million pet dogs in the United States alone. It is estimated that there is on average one dog per household in half of all American family homes. There are over 230 known pure breeds of dogs recognized by the American Kennel Club (AKC). The purpose of the AKC is to uphold the integrity dog breeds, promoting purebred dogs and breeding for type and function. Founded in 1884, the AKC advocates the purebred dog as a family companion, advancing canine health and well-being, working to protect the rights of all dog owners, and promoting responsible dog ownership.

Points to remember. There are over 230 recognized pure dog breeds.

1.2 Characteristics of Dogs

Dogs have a large variety of size ranges (height to weight). The height of dogs at the shoulder ranges from 6 to 40 inches and weight varies from 2 to over 200 pounds. Life expectancy ranges from 9 to 15 years, with some dogs now living into their early 20s. Small dogs have a longer life expectancy than large and giant breeds (Figure 1.1). Dogs share the following common traits:

- shedding hair once per year;
- non-retractable claws;
- 42 adult teeth, 28 baby teeth;
- pointed canine teeth;
- sweat glands located on nose and feet;
- panting;
- hearing two times better than in humans and at higher frequencies;

1.3 Classes of Breeds

Dog breeds are classified by the reason for their development and purpose or use. There are seven groups of dogs that have been organized based on the dog's original purpose and the traits it possesses in today's world (Table 1.1).

Points to remember. There are seven groups of dogs based on their reason for development.

1.3.1 Herding Group

The herding group developed in 1983 and is the newest AKC classification (Figure 1.2). All herding breeds share the ability to control the movement of other animals, by driving, moving, and containing livestock in specific locations. Many of these dogs will nip at the heels of animals to move them in set directions. Many herding dogs, as household pets, never cross paths with a farm animal. Nevertheless, pure instinct prompts these dogs to gently herd their owners, especially children within

Veterinary Guide to Animal Breeds, First Edition. Beth Vanhorn.
© 2018 John Wiley & Sons, Inc. Published 2018 by John Wiley & Sons, Inc.
Companion website: www.wiley.com/go/vanhorn/breeds

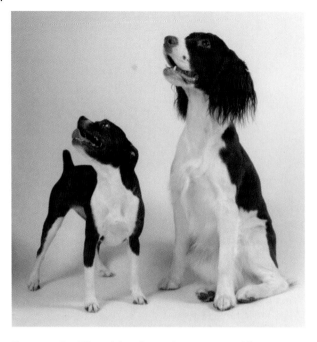

Figure 1.1 Small breed dogs have a longer average life expectancy than large and giant breeds. The larger the dog breed, the shorter the life span. *Source*: Courtesy of Shari Krause.

the family. Herding dogs are among the most intelligent, making excellent companions, and also obedience and agility dogs. Herding breeds are high in energy and bond strongly to their human companions.

Table 1.1 Groups of dogs.

Group	Breeds	Purpose
Herding	Shepherds, Collies, Sheepdogs, Corgi	Driving, moving, and containing livestock
Hound	Beagle, Greyhound, Foxhound, Bloodhound	Use of senses for hunting and tracking, such as hearing, sight, and smell
Non-sporting	Dalmatian, Bulldog, Poodle, Boston Terrier	Pets and companions
Sporting	Retrievers, Pointers, Setters, Spaniels	Active hunting by scents in the air and ground
Terrier	Airedale, Schnauzer, West Highland, Scottish	Catching and flushing out rodents and small game
Toy	Chihuahua, Pug, Pomeranian, Shih Tzu	Pets and companions
Working	Boxer, Mastiffs, St Bernard, Rottweiler	Guarding, guiding, herding and obedience

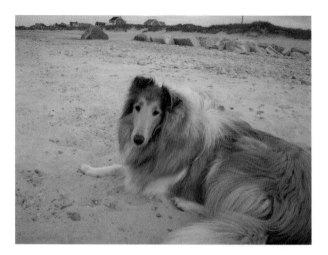

Figure 1.2 The Collie is an example of a herding group dog breed.

1.3.2 Hound Group

The hound group shares the common traits used for hunting (Figure 1.3). Some dogs have acute senses, such as smell, hearing, and sight. Others demonstrate relentless stamina as if they will run forever. The hound group is diverse, with sight hounds that are slim and built for speed and foxhounds and bloodhounds that are larger boned and built for tracking and hunting. Some hounds share the distinct ability to produce a unique barking or baying sound. Many dogs within the hound group have floppy to drooping ears.

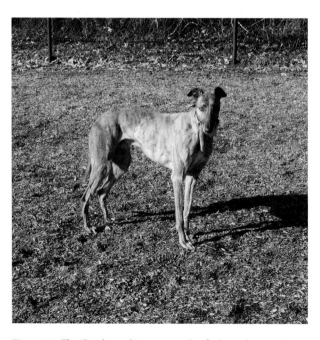

Figure 1.3 The Greyhound is an example of a hound group dog breed.

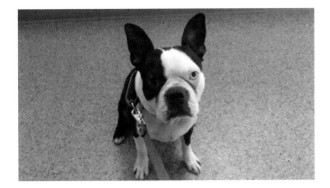

Figure 1.4 The Boston Terrier is an example of a non-sporting group dog breed. *Source*: Courtesy of Shari Krause.

1.3.3 Non-Sporting Group

The non-sporting group is another diverse group (Figure 1.4). This group used to be classified as miscellaneous and has a variety of size differences, coat types, and personalities and vary in popularity. Each breed in the non-sporting group has a specific background but most are no longer used today for their original development purposes. The non-sporting group breeds do not fit easily into other groups.

1.3.4 Sporting Group

The sporting group is naturally active, alert, and honest companion dogs used in many types of hunting sports (Figure 1.5). Known for their instincts in water and woods, many of these breeds actively continue to participate in hunting and field trial activities, and also

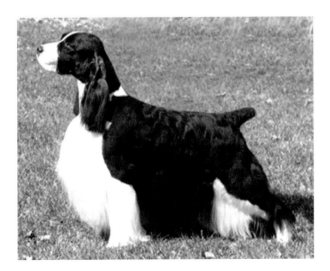

Figure 1.5 The English Springer Spaniel is an example of a sporting group dog breed. *Source*: Courtesy of Shari Krause.

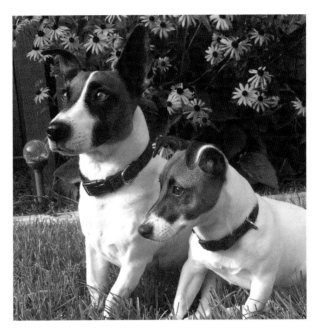

Figure 1.6 The Parson Russell Terrier is an example of a terrier group dog breed.

show obedience and agility. Sporting dogs require regular exercise and activity and human attention. The sporting group breeds include the Retrievers, Spaniels, Pointers and Setters.

1.3.5 Terrier Group

The terrier group has a wide range of sizes and personalities (Figure 1.6). The breeds are feisty, energetic dogs that typically have little tolerance for other animals, including other dogs. These breeds were bred to hunt and kill rodents and vermin. Many continue to project the attitude that they are always eager for a spirited argument. Most terriers have wiry and dense coats that require special grooming known as stripping in order to maintain a characteristic appearance. The terrier breeds are relatively smaller in size and were bred to go into dens to retrieve and flush out animals. The terriers tend to have independent personalities.

1.3.6 Toy Group

The toy group is small but mighty and often the dogs do not recognize their small stature (Figure 1.7). The toy breeds are known to be quite vocal and lively but are loving companion animals. They are popular with city dwellers and people without much living space. They make ideal apartment dogs and terrific lap dogs.

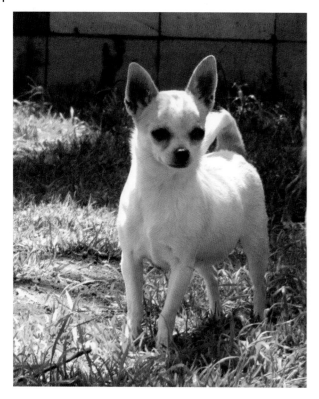

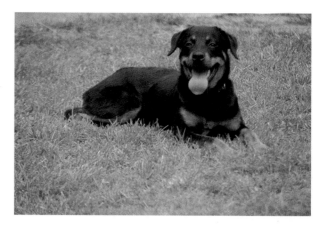

Figure 1.8 The Rottweiler is an example of a working group dog breed. *Source*: Courtesy of Kimberly Wilson.

The miscellaneous group includes dog breeds that are awaiting full approval by the AKC. The breeds on the waiting list vary from year to year and upon full approval will be assigned to the appropriate group.

Figure 1.7 The Chihuahua is an example of a toy group dog breed.

1.4 Summary

Dogs have adapted over the years through breeding and cross-breeding with a variety of breeds and characteristics. Knowledge of the classes of dogs will aid in the identification of dog breeds. It is important to remember that many purebred breeds of dogs are crossed and we are seeing more and more hybrid breeds and designer breeds that some day may be a recognized registered dog breed. Dog breed roles were focused around types of work and services for improving human lives. The vast number of activities and uses in which dogs were once involved has resulted in the formation of a wide variety of breeds. Most dogs serve a companion-type role in today's society. However, many breeds are still involved in their traditional roles.

1.3.7 Working Group

The working group was bred to perform such jobs as guarding property, pulling sleds, and performing water rescues (Figure 1.8). They have been assets to humans throughout the ages. This group of dogs are intelligent, quick to learn, capable animals that make solid companions. Their considerable size and strength alone, however, make many working dogs not suitable for all people. They require training and obedience for proper control.

Sources

American Kennel Club (AKC) (2016).
APPA (2014) *2013–2014 APPA National Pet Owners Survey*. American Pet Product Association, Greenwich, CT.
AVMA (2012) *U.S. Pet Ownership & Demographics Sourcebook*, American Veterinary Medical Association, Schaumburg, IL.

Further Reading

American Kennel Club (2015) *The New Complete Dog Book*, 21st edn., i-5 Publishing, Irvine, CA.
Bell, J.S., Cavanaugh, K.E., Tilley, L.P., and Smith, F.C.W. (2012) *Veterinary Medical Guide to Dog and Cat Breeds*, Teton NewMedia, Jackson, WY.
Coile, D.C. (2015) *Encyclopedia of Dogs*, Barron's Educational Series, Hauppauge, NY.
Edwards, R. (2016) *Cats and Dogs Encyclopedia*, CreateSpace.

2

Cat Breed Identification

OBJECTIVES

Upon completion of this chapter, the reader should be able to:

- recognize common breeds of cat species;
- identify and describe Cat Fancier's Association (CFA) recognized cat breeds;
- discuss and describe the classes of cats.

2.1 Introduction

Cats were domesticated over 2000 years ago and developed from wild, larger felines. Cats have become the most popular animal in pet ownership, with over 80 million pet cats in the United States alone. This is in part due to the less space and personal attention necessary for cat care compared with other animals. There are over 40 known pure breeds of cats recognized by the Cat Fanciers' Association (CFA). The purpose of the CFA is to promote the welfare of cats and focus on quality breed standards and promote an interest in pedigreed cats. Established in 1906, the CFA has registered over 2 million pedigreed cats. The task of cats is to serve as a hunter of rodents and vermin. The cat's naturally independent attitude is less suited for a working animal and more towards that of a pet and companion. Most cats in the United States are not registered and are of mixed breeds. In many countries, cats are considered God-like creatures and highly worshipped and considered sacred.

Points to remember. There are over 40 recognized pure breeds of cats.

2.2 Characteristics of Cats

Cats range over a wide variety of sizes, and are mostly in weight range 4–20 plus pounds (Figure 2.1). Their average life expectancy ranges from 10 to 15 years, with many now living into their early to mid-20s. Cats share the following common traits:

- retractable claws;
- 30 adult teeth, 26 baby teeth;
- pointed canine teeth;
- whiskers: vibrissae act as antennae, organ of touch and balance, catch sound reflections;
- vision: specialized night vision, can see up to 120 feet;
- hearing $1\frac{1}{2}$ times better than that of dogs, semicircular ear canals to maintain balance, ability to land on feet during falls;
- smell: 14 times better than that of humans.

2.3 Classes of Breeds

There are seven classes of cats recognized by the CFA, based on show and competition. The classes include the kitten class, which is for altered and unaltered pedigreed kittens between the ages of 4 and 8 months (Figure 2.2). The championship class is for unaltered pedigreed cats over the age of 8 months (Figure 2.3). Premiership classes are for altered pedigreed cats over 8 months of age. Veteran classes are for altered and unaltered pedigreed cats over the age of 7 years (Figure 2.4). Household pet classes are for non-pedigreed cats over 4 months of age, and if over 8 months of age must be altered and may not be declawed. The miscellaneous class is for newly recognized breeds and will then become provisional breeds once the CFA has stated that they are considered a pedigreed cat.

Veterinary Guide to Animal Breeds, First Edition. Beth Vanhorn.
© 2018 John Wiley & Sons, Inc. Published 2018 by John Wiley & Sons, Inc.
Companion website: www.wiley.com/go/vanhorn/breeds

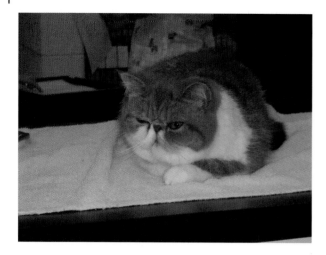

Figure 2.1 An example of a purebred cat breed.

2.3.1 Hair Coat Types

Cats may also be categorized by their hair coat type. Cats may be long hair, short hair, and hairless (Figure 2.5). See Table 2.1 as an example. Cat hair lengths are variable and in some breeds the length of hair may be difficult to distinguish owing to the coat texture and thickness.

> **Points to remember.** Cat hair coats come in three types: long hair, short hair, and hairless.

2.3.2 Color Variations

There are many coat color variations that can be mistaken for different cat breeds. As each cat breed has a specific color, some domestic cats of unknown breeds can

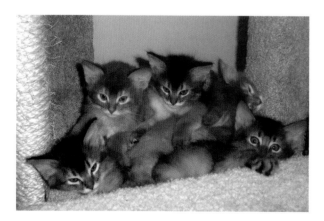

Figure 2.2 An example of a kitten class entry between 4 and 8 months of age.

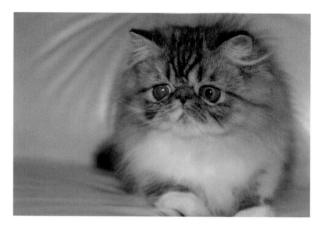

Figure 2.3 An example of a championship class entry.

have a variety of different colors. Many color terms are associated with cats. The term "tabby" is used to describe a coat pattern with varied striping over a base color (Figure 2.6). Calico is a mixture of black, brown, and orange hairs in a dark shading and are typically female cats (Figure 2.7). Tortoiseshell is also a mixture of black, brown, and orange hairs in a variable pattern in a lighter shade and is also typically a female cat (Figure 2.8). Diluted colors are also seen as a pale version of the darker color. Bicolor patterns refer to a white background coat with a solid patched darker color pattern. Parti-color refers to one color superimposed on a white background.

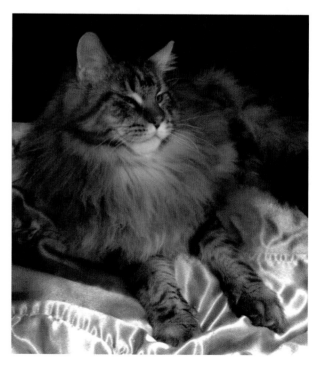

Figure 2.4 An example of a veteran class entry.

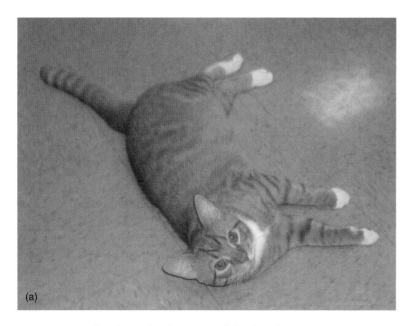

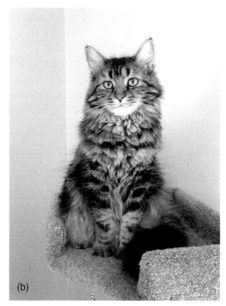

Figure 2.5 Examples of (a) a short hair coat and (b) a long hair coat.

Table 2.1 Types of hair coats.

Type	Breeds	Description
Long hair	Persian, Himalayan, Ragdoll	Long, thick, hair coat with increased shedding
Short hair	Siamese, Burmese, Russian Blue	Smooth, thin, hair coat with moderate shedding
Hairless	Sphynx	No hair or almost no hair over the majority of the body

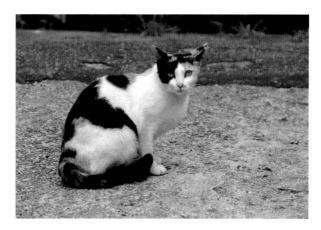

Figure 2.7 An example of a calico color hair coat.

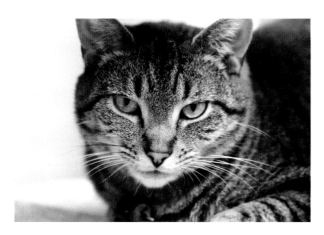

Figure 2.6 An example of a tabby color hair coat.

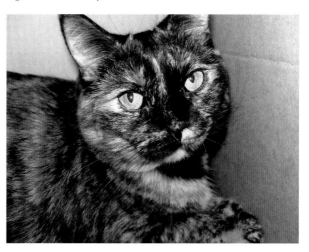

Figure 2.8 An example of a tortoiseshell hair coat.

2.4 Summary

Many cat breeds have developed from cross-breeding and many cats have developed genetic defects that have made their characteristics favorable, hence continued breeding for these mutations has continued and developed into a cat breed. For example, American Curls and Scottish Folds have genetic mutations to their specific ear set. Many non-pedigreed cats may have characteristics resembling purebreds, but without known parentage they are based on their hair length and may be described as domestic shorthairs or longhairs. Knowledge of the classes of cats will aid in the identification of cat breeds. In the United States, most cats are of mixed-breed descent but may be easily recognized by some purebred characteristics.

Sources

Cat Fanciers' Association (2016).

APPA (2014) *2013–2014 APPA National Pet Owners Survey.* American Pet Product Association, Greenwich, CT.

AVMA (2012) *U.S. Pet Ownership & Demographics Sourcebook*, American Veterinary Medical Association, Schaumburg, IL.

Further Reading

Bell, J.S., Cavanaugh, K.E., Tilley, L.P., and Smith, F.C.W. (2012) *Veterinary Medical Guide to Dog and Cat Breeds*, Teton NewMedia, Jackson, WY.

Dennis-Bryan, K. (ed.) (2013) *The Complete Cat Breed Book*, DK Publishing, New York.

Edwards, R. (2016) *Cats and Dogs Encylopedia*, CreateSpace.

3

Rabbit Breed Identification

OBJECTIVES

Upon completion of this chapter, the reader should be able to:

- recognize common breeds of rabbit species;
- identify and describe American Rabbit Breeders Association (ARBA) recognized rabbit breeds;
- discuss and describe the five types of rabbits.

3.1 Introduction

Rabbit breeds developed and were domesticated from wild European rabbits and hares. There are approximately 45 rabbit breeds officially recognized by the American Rabbits Breeders Association (ARBA). The purpose of the ARBA is to promote, develop, and improve domesticated rabbit breeds. The rabbits may be cross-bred to create mixed-breed rabbits. Most of the breeds originally developed for one of four purposes: meat, pelt, wool, or show. Many rabbit breeds can make a good pet. There are two factors to take into consideration when selecting a rabbit breed: the size of the rabbit and the amount of care that it requires. Rabbits have become a very popular small animal pet in the last several years. Rabbits are mammals classified as lagomorphs.

Points to remember. There are approximately 45 recognized rabbit breeds.

3.2 Characteristics of Rabbits

Rabbits range in size, color, and hair coat types, and vary in weight from 2 to over 16 pounds. They are mammals with long ears, short, fluffy tails, and powerful, large hind legs that allow movement by hopping (Figure 3.1). Rabbits share the following characteristics:

- long, large ears;
- long, powerful, and muscular hind legs;
- large, round eyes.

Rabbits have four toes on their hind feet that are long and webbed to keep them from spreading apart as they jump. Their front feet have five toes each. Some species of rabbit can reach speeds of 35–45 miles per hour. Rabbits have two pairs of sharp incisors (front teeth), one pair at the top and the other at the bottom, making a total of four, whereas rodents have two incisors. They also have two peg teeth, also called wolf teeth, located behind the top incisors. Their teeth are specifically adapted for gnawing and grow continuously throughout their lives. Rabbits have 28 adult teeth. Hair coats come in a variety of lengths and textures, from smooth to extremely long and fine hair that requires large amounts of grooming. Hares are a larger version of the rabbit and are in the same family (Figure 3.2). They have longer ears, do not build nests as rabbits do, and live above ground rather than digging tunnels like rabbits. Rabbits are coprophagic, which means that they eat their own feces, and pass two types of feces. Firm, dry, pelleted feces are passed during the daytime and soft, moist, night feces are passed during the night; these are rich in vitamins and proteins and are eaten shortly after being passed.

3.3 Types of Rabbits

Rabbits are classified by five types of body structures: small commercial, commercial, semi-arch, full arch, and cylindrical (Table 3.1).

Points to remember. There are five classes of rabbits based on size and body shape.

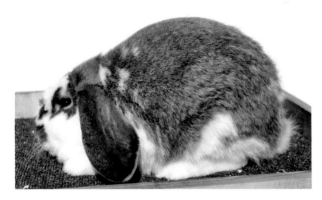

Figure 3.1 Example of a rabbit. *Source*: Courtesy of Wendy MacDonald.

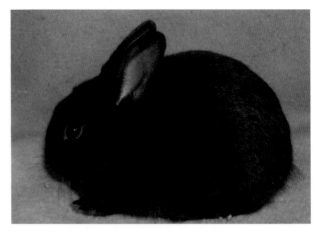

Figure 3.3 Example of a small commercial type rabbit breed. *Source*: Courtesy of Wendy MacDonald.

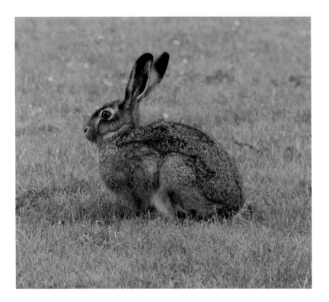

Figure 3.2 Example of a hare.

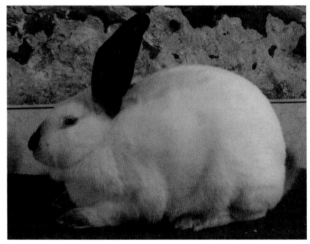

Figure 3.4 Example of a commercial type rabbit breed.

Table 3.1 Classes of rabbits.

Class	Breeds	Characteristics
Small commercial	Polish, Holland Lop, Netherland Dwarf	Dwarf and miniature; 2–7 pounds
Standard commercial	New Zealand, Rex	Medium size, 8–12 pounds
Semi-arch	American, American Chinchilla	Large size, 12–14 pounds, with slightly rounded back
Full-arch	Giant Angora, Giant Chinchilla, Flemish Giant	Giant size, over 14 pounds, with rounded back
Cylindrical	Californian	Long, slim, cylinder-shaped body

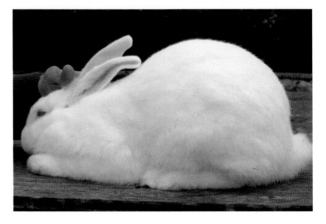

Figure 3.5 Example of a semi-arch type rabbit breed. *Source*: Courtesy of Wendy MacDonald.

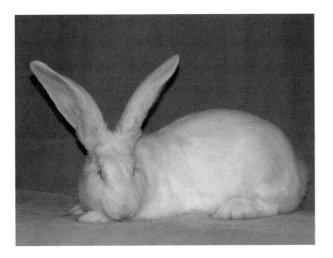

Figure 3.6 Example of a full arch type rabbit breed.

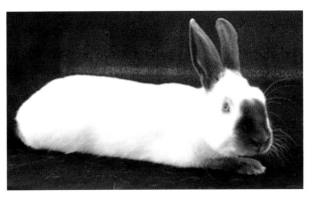

Figure 3.7 Example of a cylindrical type rabbit breed.

3.4 Summary

Rabbits have been raised for meat, pelts, hair, and by-products and as pets. Breeding domestic rabbits can be rewarding and profitable. A rabbit kept as a pet may be exhibited in shows or can be a good source of meat. Raising and owning rabbits is enjoyable and exciting. It can be done in any location with just a small amount of land. As domestic pets, rabbits are perfect to raise and own: they do not make any noise, need little living space, and require small amounts of food and water. Rabbits are also used as important tools in infectious disease research, toxin and antitoxin development, and vaccine research. Rabbit wool also has a profitable value. Rabbit wool may be dyed, dressed, sheared, and made into clothing and bedding products. Knowledge of the types of rabbit body structures will help aid in the identification of specific breeds.

The most common body types are the small commercial and commercial types (Figure 3.3). Small commercial rabbit types include dwarf and miniature sizes that weigh between 2 and 7 pounds. They are popular pets and have quiet dispositions. Commercial breeds are medium-sized breeds with weights between 8 and 12 pounds (Figure 3.4). Semi-arch type rabbits are large breeds ranging in body size from 12 to 14 pounds with a slight back curvature (Figure 3.5) and full arch types are giant-size breeds weighing over 14 pounds that have a rounded appearance to their back (Figure 3.6). Cylindrical types are long and thin, with a cylinder shape to their bodies (Figure 3.7).

Sources

American Rabbit Breeders Association (2016).

AVMA (2012) *U.S. Pet Ownership & Demographics Sourcebook*, American Veterinary Medical Association, Schaumburg, IL.

Further Reading

Stone, L.M. (2016) *Rabbit Breeds: The Pocket Guide to 49 Essential Breeds*, Storey Publishing, North Adams, MA.

Whitman, B.D. (2004) *Domestic Rabbits & Their Histories: Breeds of the World*, Leathers Publishing, Overland Park, KS.

4

Guinea Pig Breed Identification

<table>
<tr><td>

OBJECTIVES

Upon completion of this chapter, the reader should be able to:

- recognize common breeds of guinea pigs;
- identify and describe American Rabbit Breeders Association (ARBA) and American Cavy Breeders Association (ACBA) recognized guinea pig breeds;
- discuss and describe the types of guinea pigs.

</td></tr>
</table>

4.1 Introduction

Guinea pigs originated in South America, where they were raised for thousands of years as a source of meat. The guinea pig, also called the cavy, is a member of the rodent family and related to chinchillas. The American Rabbit Breeders Association (ARBA) was founded for the purpose of the development, promotion, and improvement of the domestic rabbit and cavy. The American Cavy Breeders Association was further developed to focus on the development and improvement of the cavy as a pet, exhibition, and research animal. There are over 10 different recognized breeds of guinea pigs.

> **Points to remember.** There are over 10 different breeds of guinea pigs.

4.2 Characteristics of Guinea Pigs

The guinea pig is a short-legged, large-bodied animal with small ears (Figure 4.1). Guinea pigs share the following common traits:

- stout bodied;
- short limbs;
- small ears;
- tailless.

Guinea pigs may have short or long hair or be hairless and come in a variety of colors and combinations of patterns. Guinea pigs are large in terms of rodent species, weighing from 1.5 to 2.5 pounds and with lengths of 8–10 inches. They are very social animals, with vocal chattering, whistling, and chirping sounds. Guinea pigs tend to be gentle pets that are docile and easy to handle. The male is larger than the female and they have very sensitive senses of hearing and smell. Guinea pigs have four digits on the front feet and three digits on the hind feet. Guinea pigs cannot synthesize vitamin C as most other animals can and therefore must have vitamin C supplemented in their diet. They have 20 adult teeth that are open rooted and ever growing. They are herbivores that eat a lot of roughage material for proper digestion and should not have a variety of different foods as this can be disruptive to their digestive tracts. Female pubic bones will begin to fuse at around 6 months of age if not previously bred. This fusion can lead to dystocia and potential death of the guinea pig during labor.

4.3 Types of Guinea Pigs

The Abyssinian guinea pig is a breed recognized by its unique hair pattern that forms many rosettes or cowlicks that create swirls throughout the coat (Figure 4.2). The American guinea pig is the most popular breed and has a short, dense, straight hair coat (Figure 4.2). The Coronet breed is characterized by a long lock of hair on the top of the head. The Himalayan breed is marked similarly to the cat breed and is considered albino with a darker color of points, usually black markings, over the ears, nose, and feet. The Peruvian guinea pig has uniform long hair over the entire body and the hair coat can grow to lengths of several inches (Figure 4.3). The Rex is a short-hair breed with hair less than 1 cm in length and has three different types of hair to protect its coat that give it a wool-like appearance. The Silkie is similar to the Peruvian in that it has a longer hair coat that is soft and silky. The hair over the face is short and the long hair coat is slicked back over

Veterinary Guide to Animal Breeds, First Edition. Beth Vanhorn.
© 2018 John Wiley & Sons, Inc. Published 2018 by John Wiley & Sons, Inc.
Companion website: www.wiley.com/go/vanhorn/breeds

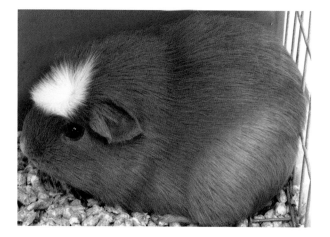

Figure 4.1 Example of a guinea pig.

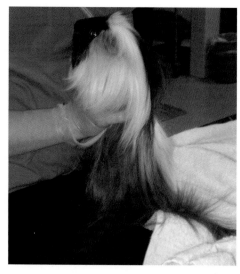

Figure 4.3 Example of a Peruvian guinea pig.

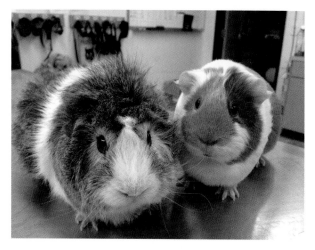

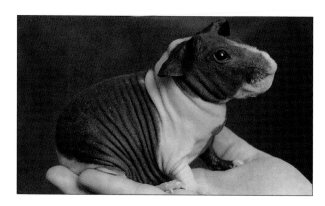

Figure 4.2 Examples of an Abyssinian guinea pig (left) and an American guinea pig (right).

Figure 4.4 Example of a skinny hairless guinea pig.

the top of the head and entire body. The skinny guinea pig is hairless but may develop a few hairs on the legs or feet (Figure 4.4). The Teddy breed has a short, kinky hair coat that has a wiry texture. The Texel has a soft, curly hair coat over the entire body. The White Crested has a short-hair coat that is marked with a white spot on top of the head called a crest.

4.4 Summary

The guinea pig is a small rodent often kept as a pet or for show and comes in a variety of sizes, colors, and hair types. They tend to be very gentle and relatively easy to care for. Knowledge of the different types of breeds will help in identification of the guinea pig.

Sources

American Rabbit Breeders Association (2016).
AVMA (2012) *U.S. Pet Ownership & Demographics Sourcebook*, American Veterinary Medical Association, Schaumburg, IL.

Further Reading

Gurney, P. (1999) *What's My Guinea Pig? A Guide to Guinea Pig Breeds*, Tfh Publications, Neptune City, NJ.

5

Pocket Pet Breed Identification

<table>
<tr><td>

OBJECTIVES

Upon completion of this chapter, the reader should be able to:

- recognize common breeds of pocket pet species, including mice, rats, and hamsters;
- recognize and identify common species of pocket pets, including chinchillas, hedgehogs, ferrets, and gerbils;
- identify and describe associations, groups, and clubs that recognize breeds of pocket pet species.

</td></tr>
</table>

5.1 Introduction

The American Fancy Mouse and Rat Association (AFMRA) was founded in 1983 with the purpose of promoting and encouraging the breeding and exhibition of fancy rats and mice and also of educating the public on their positive qualities as companion animals and providing information on their proper care. The Rat and Mouse Club of America (RMFA) was founded to promote the proper care and handling of rats and mice, and also responsible breeding and hobby growth. The National Hamster Council (NHC) was established in 1949 and is the oldest hamster organization in the world recognizing the interests of owning, showing and breeding hamsters. The National Gerbil Society (NGS), developed in 1970, promotes gerbils for showing and raising as pets. The Chinchilla Breeders Organization (CBO) was developed in 1999 as a place for chinchilla owners and breeders to come together to learn, share, and grow. The International Hedgehog Association (IHA) was formed with the purpose of educating the public in the care and betterment of hedgehogs and to facilitate the rescue, welfare, promotion, and care of hedgehogs. The American Ferret Association (AFA) was developed in 1987 as a way to promote and protect ferrets and provide information to ferret owners and

enthusiasts. Each of these groups collectively has one overall goal in mind: to promote, educate, and preserve the small animals that many people have kept as pets and as companions for numerous years. Many pocket pet species are classified in the rodent family.

Points to remember. The term "pocket pet" refers to a small domesticated animal kept as a pet and is typically of a size that would be able to fit in a person's pocket.

5.2 Characteristics of Mice

Adult mice typically weigh about 1 ounce and are approximately 2.5–3.5 inches long, not including the tail (Figure 5.1). Male mice are typically larger than females. Pet mice are available in many colors and coat patterns owing to specialized breeding. Coats can be smooth, curly, long-haired or a combination. The most common color variations include brown, black, tan, gray, and albino, also with lighter and darker shades of these. House mice were domesticated around 1800 by both Europeans and Asians. The best known species of mouse is the common house mouse (*Mus musculus*).

Mice have a pointed nose, a split upper lip, and 16 adult teeth. They have a great field of vision as their eyes are on the side of their head but their detailed vision is poor. They have well-developed, large ears for hearing and an acute sense of smell. Mice are best housed with other mice and are primarily nocturnal. Mice are extremely active and constantly on the move as they have a high metabolic rate.

5.3 Characteristics of Rats

There are two species of rats that have been domesticated as pets and used in research: the black rat and the brown rat. The brown rat, also known as the Norway rat, was

Veterinary Guide to Animal Breeds, First Edition. Beth Vanhorn.
© 2018 John Wiley & Sons, Inc. Published 2018 by John Wiley & Sons, Inc.
Companion website: www.wiley.com/go/vanhorn/breeds

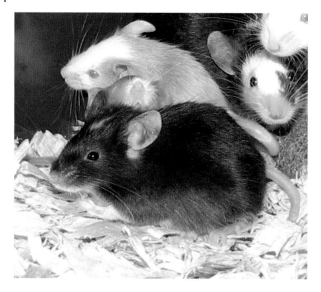

Figure 5.1 Example of a pet mouse.

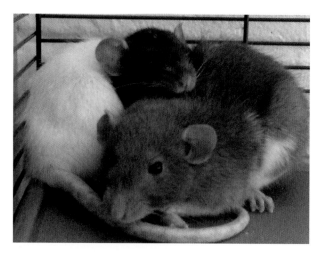

Figure 5.2 Example of a pet rat.

found on the streets of cities and in the fields of rural areas. The Norway rat became domesticated in Victorian times and people began to breed them selectively for their fur and color variety. It is believed to have originated in Asia. The black rat is thought to have originated in southern Asia and is believed to be the reservoir of the Black Plague in Europe in the early 1200s. Adult female and male rats typically weigh 12–16 and 16–23 ounces, respectively. Rats are about 9–11 inches long, not including the tail. Male rats are usually larger than females. Pet rats are available in several colors and coat patterns owing to specialized breeding (Figure 5.2). The common color variations include brown, black, tan, gray, and white, also with lighter and darker shades. Some of the more exotic colors include blue, silver, lilac, cinnamon, pearl, lynx, silver agouti, and blaze. Rex rats have a curly coat. Tailless rats are born with no tails and hairless rats have no fur. Rats can be differentiated from mice as they are larger in size and have more rows of scales on their tails. Rats have 16 teeth that are constantly erupting incisors and they are primarily nocturnal. Rats are social animals and natural burrowers. When stressed or sick, red tears can overflow from the Harderian gland within the lacrimal duct and create a red stain on the nose and face.

5.4 Characteristics of Hamsters

Hamsters are rodents and are distant relatives of mice and rats. Hamsters originated in the desert areas of Syria and the Middle East. Adult Golden hamsters, also known as Syrian hamsters, are approximately 6–8 inches

in length and weigh 6–7 ounces (Figure 5.3). Females are usually larger than males and also tend to be more aggressive. All domesticated hamsters are descendants of the Golden hamster. Most other varieties of hamsters are slightly smaller and weigh less. A unique feature of hamsters is the outpouching of the cheeks on both sides of the mouth that extends along the sides of the head and neck all the way back to the shoulders. In the wild, these large pouches allow hamsters to gather food during foraging trips that they then carry back to their nest to store and later consume. Pet owners who suddenly see a fully distended pouch for the first time may fear their pet has some sort of fast-growing tumor or swelling, but this is not the case. A female can also pack a whole litter of newborns into her cheek pouches to move them to another location. Another unusual characteristic of hamsters is paired glands in the skin over the flanks. These

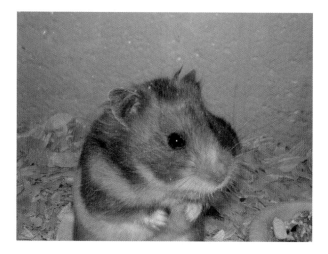

Figure 5.3 Example of a pet hamster.

glands appear as dark spots within the hair coat, and are much more obvious in males than in females. Hamsters use these glands to mark their territory. Hamsters are nocturnal and active at night. Hamsters have almost no tail and their skin is loose and pliable. They have 16 adult teeth that grow continuously. Hamsters can go into a hibernation state if the temperature drops below about 46 °F (8 °C) and have a decreased body temperature, heart rate, and respiratory rate for several days. Hamsters are sound sleepers and when startled from sleep often bite.

5.5 Characteristics of Chinchillas

Chinchillas are members of the rodent family. They originated in the Andes Mountains of South America. During the eighteenth century, chinchillas were hunted for their fur and faced extinction until laws banned hunting them. Today there are about 3000 ranches throughout the United States and Canada that breed chinchillas, and they are increasingly popular as pets. Chinchillas have a very thick coat of fur, with as many as 60 follicles per hair, and the hair coat is exceptionally soft as there are fewer guard hairs than in other pocket pets (Figure 5.4). Their original blue–gray color has now been developed with coats that are black, gray, white, beige, and combinations of each. Their thick fur not only keeps them warm but also protects them from parasites and predators. Chinchillas clean their fur by rolling in dust and they also have the ability to release fur as a defense mechanism: if one is grabbed roughly by a predator or handler, it will leave a patch of fur behind. Chinchillas have a rounded body, large mouse-like ears, short legs, long whiskers, and a long, bushy, squirrel-like tail. A newborn chinchilla weighs 2–2.5 ounces and an adult's weight ranges from

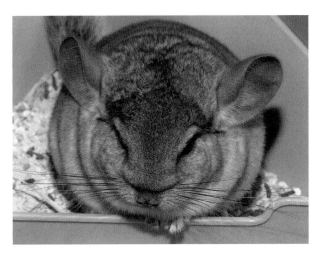

Figure 5.4 Example of a pet chinchilla.

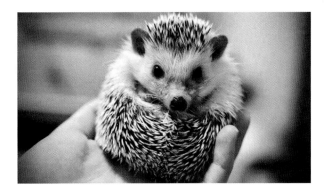

Figure 5.5 Example of a pet hedgehog.

1 to 1.5 pounds. Females are usually larger than males. They can grow to be 10 inches long, with a tail that can add a further 6 inches at full maturity. They have 20 adult teeth that are open rooted and grow continuously. They are nocturnal. Chinchillas are very active, agile and like to jump; however, they are rather shy.

5.6 Characteristics of Hedgehogs

Hedgehogs are distant relatives of shrews and resemble shrews in the face by having a long, pointy snout. The average hedgehog weighs approximately $\frac{1}{2}$–$1\frac{1}{4}$ pounds and most are the size of a softball or slightly larger when they are rolled into a ball. Some adult hedgehogs have a slightly larger build and can weigh up to 2 pounds. Most hedgehogs are 6–8 inches in length, but it is difficult to measure a hedgehog accurately and consistently because their body changes shape when it is balled up, relaxed, sitting, or moving. A hedgehog has spines covering its outer body and back as a way of protection (Figure 5.5). The spines do not release like in a porcupine. About 35% of the hedgehog's weight is the spines. Hedgehogs have an orbicularis muscle that contracts like a drawstring to allow it to roll up into a ball. A small tail is tucked up under its spines.

5.7 Characteristics of Gerbils

Domesticated gerbils originated in the deserts of North Africa and Central Asia and are sometimes referred to as Mongolian gerbils or jirds. Gerbils are relatives of mice and rats and have been bred as pets since the 1960s. They are burrowing rodents with short bodies and have a hunched appearance (Figure 5.6). Gerbils are known for their curious and mild temperament. Gerbils are very social creatures and do best when kept in pairs. Adult gerbils weigh 2–3 ounces. Males are slightly larger than

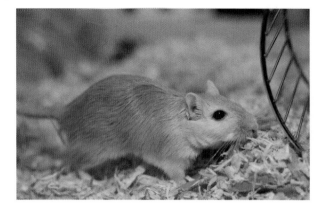

Figure 5.6 Example of a pet gerbil.

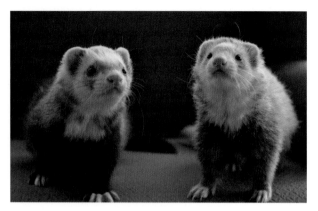

Figure 5.7 Example of a pet ferret.

females. The coats of gerbils in the wild are agouti colored, with a mix of gray, yellow, and black, and with an off-white stomach. Breeding has produced gerbils with many different coat colors, including black, buff, white, gray, and spotted. They are about the size of mice, with their bodies measuring about 4 inches in length; their fur-covered tails can add an additional 3 inches at maturity. The tail has a bushy tip that is used for support while standing. Gerbils have a ventral marking gland on their abdomen. The gland appears as an orange–tan hairless area that is usually oval in shape. In male gerbils, the gland enlarges during puberty and produces an oily secretion. Male gerbils may use this as a way of marking territory, and they can sometimes be seen rubbing their abdomen on objects. They have 16 adult teeth and an enlarged adrenal gland that allows them to conserve water.

5.8 Characteristics of Ferrets

Ferrets developed from the black-footed ferret and now in domestication are bred for a variety of over 30 colors, including black, white, and sable. The domestic ferret is part of the Mustelidae animal family that includes weasels, badgers, and minks. However, unlike these wild species, they are fully domesticated and would not survive outside captivity. Ferrets have been in captivity for more than 2000 years and have become popular pets over the last decade in the United States. Ferrets were originally used as hunting animals to help control rabbits and rodents and then were raised for their pelts. Keeping domestic ferrets as pets is not legal in all US states. A ferret is a small mammal, usually weighing less than 5 pounds. Females weigh 1.5–2 pounds at maturity and are much smaller than males, which usually weigh at least 3 pounds and occasionally grow as heavy as 7 pounds.

Ferrets are curious and determined, with thin, long, and slinky bodies, and are quite the entertainers that can easily get them in a lot of trouble! (Figure 5.7). They have flexible spines that allow for agility, climbing, and jumping. Their long tails are about half the length of their body and head. Ferrets have scent glands that produce a musky odor even after being de-scented and have sebaceous secretions in their skin that also produce a musky odor. Ferrets have 40 adult teeth that include very sharp canine teeth, are primarily nocturnal, and do not see well in bright light. Ferrets have highly developed senses of touch, smell, and hearing. They have especially thick skin over their neck and shoulders. They experience seasonal changes in body fat, losing weight in the summer and gaining weight back in the winter. They shed their hair in the spring and fall. Their claws are not retractable and require regular trimming. Ferrets are highly susceptible to canine distemper and must be vaccinated against the virus as it is typically fatal in ferrets. Ferrets are also inclined to develop the human influenza virus. It is important for female ferret owners to be alerted that unspayed females will remain in their estrus cycle if they are not bred and can develop estrogen toxicity with bone marrow suppression and can have internal bleeding and severe anemia.

5.9 Summary

Pocket pets have become highly sought after as pets for both children and adults. They are small and relatively easy to care for, with minimal space requirements. However, some more exotic species may require specialized care and understanding. Basic descriptions and characteristics can help identify the different breeds and species of common pocket pets.

Sources

American Fancy Mouse and Rat Association (AFMRA) (2016).

American Ferret Association (AFA) (2016).

Chinchilla Breeders Organization (CBO) (2016).

International Hedgehog Association (IHA) (2016).

National Gerbil Society (NGS) (2016).

National Hamster Council (NHC) (2016).

Rat and Mouse Club of America (RMFA) (2016).

AVMA (2012) *U.S. Pet Ownership & Demographics Sourcebook*, American Veterinary Medical Association, Schaumburg, IL.

Alderton, D. (2016) *The Illustrated Practical Guide to Small Pets and Pet Care*, Anness Publishing, London.

Bartlett, P. (2015) *The Hamster Handbook*, Barron's Educational Series, Hauppauge, NY.

Delaney, S. (2014) *Gerbils: the Ultimate Guide to Gerbil Care*, Amazon Digital Services.

Huggins, J. (2010) *The Chinchilla Breeder's Diary*, CreateSpace.

Mossop, W.J. (2014) *Ferrets: Their Care and Handling*, CreateSpace.

Pellham, K.H. (2015) *Hedgehog Care*, CreateSpace.

Yee, S. (2015) *Chinchilla Care Handbook*, Amazon Digital Services.

Further Reading

AFRMA (2012) *AFRMA Breeding Rats and Mice: Care and Guidelines*, 6th edn., American Fancy Rat and Mouse Association, Riverside, CA.

6

Avian Breed Identification

6.1 Introduction

Birds are becoming an increasingly popular pet and can be excellent companion animals (Figure 6.1). Birds, also known as avians, come in a variety of sizes, colors, and personalities. Birds vary in many ways in that some have the ability to sing, talk with an extensive vocabulary, learn tricks, and complete complex tasks. Birds, however, are a large responsibility, as many species have specific needs and care requirements and, in some cases, may even outlive humans. It is important for any prospective bird owner to research and learn about a bird species before acquiring a pet bird.

The Minnesota Companion Bird Association (MCBA) was founded in 1977 as a club to promote success, education, and preserving the foundation of common companion bird species. It is also highly involved in conservation and appreciation of the rainforests and tropical environments of many species of birds in their natural habitat. Many companion bird species are not native to the locations at which they are kept and come from foreign countries, and may experience temperatures that they are not naturally accustomed to living in.

6.2 Characteristics of Companion Birds

There are more than 9500 species of avian in the world, ranging from tiny hummingbirds to large ratites, and flightless birds that are too large to fly, such as the ostrich. Companion birds can have a long lifespan; many of the larger breeds outlive humans with average life expectancies over 80 years (Figure 6.2).Companion birds share the following common traits:

- feathers that molt;
- two wings;
- two limbs with digits;
- beak;
- ability to fly depending on breed/species;
- ability to speak depending on breed/species;
- egg layers;
- hollow bones within skeleton.

Birds have heightened senses and are very similar to humans when it comes to their senses. While their front limbs are wings and their feet, beaks, and tongues have taken on many tasks for which we use our hands, birds make use of their appendages for interaction with their environment. A bird uses its beak as an additional appendage to assist with communication, mobility and movement, and social interactions, such as grooming. Birds also have a variety of vocal noise and speaking abilities. Some birds have a melodious sound with their singing whereas others make a loud screaming or screeching sound that can cause ear pain and damage. Yet others may develop a speech facility that can rival humans in talking ability and sound mimicking.

Birds kept as pets come in sizes from tiny finches that are only 4 inches from the beak to the end of their tail feathers to the large wing spans of parrots that can easily reach 40 inches. Birds have also adapted into many colorful and non-colorful hues from dull grays and browns to brilliant reds, yellows, greens, and blues (Figure 6.3). Because they are specially adapted for flight, most birds weigh very little. Even the largest parrots rarely exceed about 2.5 pounds, and medium-sized parrots may weigh from $\frac{1}{2}$ to 2 pounds. Their bones are particularly light, being hollow, and some are filled with air. A bird's wings and feathers allow for flight in most species. Each bird has a specific wing shape for its environment and living

Veterinary Guide to Animal Breeds, First Edition. Beth Vanhorn.
© 2018 John Wiley & Sons, Inc. Published 2018 by John Wiley & Sons, Inc.
Companion website: www.wiley.com/go/vanhorn/breeds

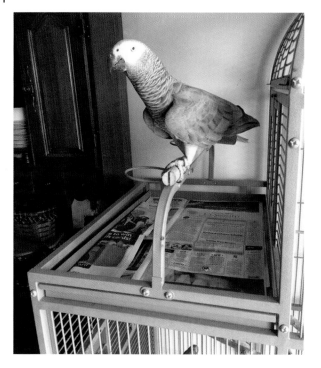

Figure 6.1 Companion birds have become increasingly popular pets.

patterns. Birds have a sensitive skin that allows them to feel and sense pressure, heat, and cold. The feathers of a bird grow from the inner layer of skin. Feathers provide assistance in flight, insulation from cold, are waterproof, and in some birds provide camouflage. In some species,

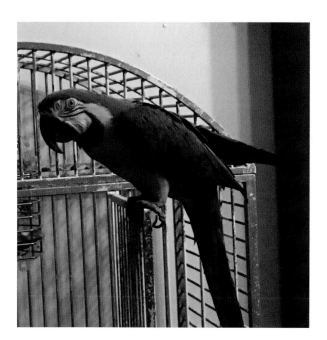

Figure 6.2 Large companion bird breeds can outlive humans.

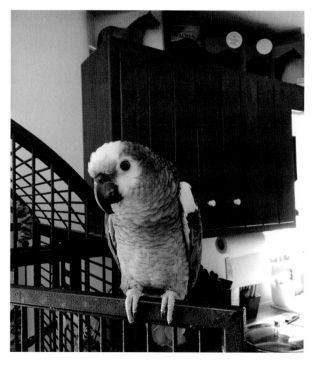

Figure 6.3 Companion birds come in a variety of colors and sizes.

the feathers can also indicate sex and mating status (Figure 6.4).

> ***Points to remember.*** There are over 9500 recognized companion bird breeds.

6.3 Orders of Companion Birds

Bird species are divided into Old World and New World species. The Old World species are primarily native to South and Central America and are fewer in number. These species are older in domestication and also include

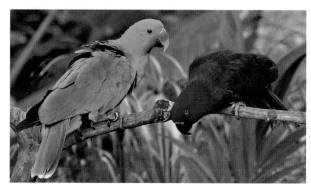

Figure 6.4 The Eclectus parrot's gender is easily identified by color differences.

Table 6.1 Bird orders.

Order	Type of birds	Species
Passerine	Perching birds, song birds	Canary, finch
Psittacine	Parrots	Amazons, macaws, cockatoos

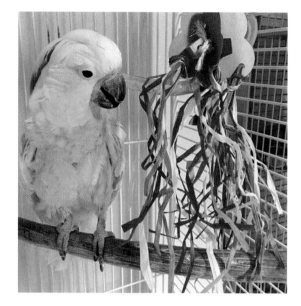

Figure 6.6 Example of a Psittacine order: the cockatoo.

the large ratites, such as the emu, rhea, and ostrich. The New World species are larger in number and include the majority of companion birds found as pets today. Many of these species are newly domesticated and in some cases are only a few generations out of the wild. Birds are not divided into breeds but into orders (Table 6.1).

The order Passerine is the largest of the orders, containing more than 50% of bird species. Most songbirds are found in this order, including canaries and finches (Figure 6.5). Passerine species have three forward-facing toes and one rear-facing toe. The beaks are pointed or slightly curved.

The order Psittacine includes more than 300 species and many of the common companion birds found in this order. Psittacines have strong, curved beaks, two forward-facing toes and two rear-facing toes. The order Psittacine includes African grays, Amazons, parakeets, cockatiels, cockatoos and conures (Figure 6.6, Figure 6.7). They are often referred to as hookbills owing to their upper beak being curved.

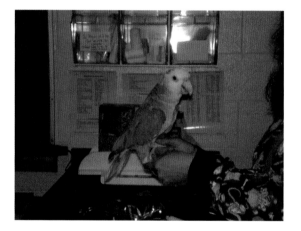

Figure 6.7 Example of a Psittacine order: the Yellow Head Amazon.

Points to remember. Companion birds are divided into two orders or groups.

Figure 6.5 Example of a Passerine order: the canary.

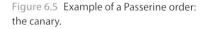

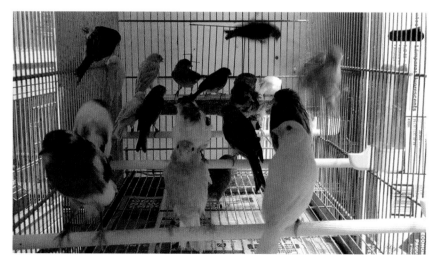

6.4 Summary

Birds have become the third most popular companion animal kept as pets in the United States. Each species has significant differences and needs, and requires thorough research before a specific bird is acquired. There are many sizes, colors, and characteristics of bird species from which to select. Many birds can live upwards of 100 years and require a lifelong commitment.

Sources

The Minnesota Companion Bird Association (MCBA) (2016).

AVMA (2012) *U.S. Pet Ownership & Demographics Sourcebook*, American Veterinary Medical Association, Schaumburg, IL.

Further Reading

Alderton, D. (2016) *A Complete Practical Guide to Caged and Aviary Birds*, Anness Publishing, London.

Gallerstein, G.A. (2003) *The Complete Pet Bird Owners Handbook*, Avian Publications, Minneapolis, MN.

7

Reptile Species Identification

7.1 Introduction

Reptiles come in a variety of sizes, shapes, and level of needs, including some reptiles that are venomous and should not be housed as traditional pets. The class *Reptilia* includes over 8000 different species; however, only a few are kept as companion pets. Reptiles include snakes, lizards, turtles, tortoise, alligators and crocodiles. The American Reptile Association (ARA) was founded as an organization for members who wanted to share their passion for reptiles. Its mission is *"To advocate education, conservation, safe handling, and the proper keeping of all reptiles."* The Society for the Study of Amphibians and Reptiles (SSAR) was established in 1958 to advance research, conservation, and education concerning amphibians and reptiles. It is the largest international herpetological society, and is recognized worldwide for having the most diverse program of publications, meetings, and other activities.

Points to remember. Reptiles include snakes, lizards, turtles, tortoises, alligators, and crocodiles.

7.2 Characteristics of Reptiles

Reptiles are vertebrates with organ systems similar to those of mammals. However, they are ectothermic and rely on environmental temperature and behavior to control their core body temperature. Reptiles share the following characteristics:

- cold blooded/ectothermic;
- scales or scutes;
- vertebrates;
- ear holes;
- four limbs or no limbs.

All reptiles exhibit ecdysis, a normal process by which the outer skin is periodically shed (see Figure 7.1). The frequency of ecdysis depends on species, age, nutritional status, environmental temperature and humidity, reproductive status, parasite load, hormonal balance, bacterial/fungal skin disease, and skin damage. The entire process can take 7–14 days. Reptiles have a tough, dry skin that is covered with scales made of keratin (Figure 7.2). The outermost layer of skin is shed regularly, but whether it sheds all at once, as in snakes, or in pieces, as in lizards, is dependent on species.

Reptiles are not considered highly social creatures, and males can become aggressive. Most companion reptile species are kept alone. The lifespan of many reptiles can exceed 10–20 years, requiring a long-term commitment from owners. Fertilization occurs internally and reptiles may lay eggs or bear live young. Many reptile species are covered in a protective layer of scales. Reptiles are either venomous or non-venomous and care should be taken to determine which species are poisonous. Reptile species that have shells covered in scutes, or bony plates, that serve as protection will often hide within their shell when frightened. It is also important to note that all reptiles naturally harbor *Salmonella* bacteria on the

Veterinary Guide to Animal Breeds, First Edition. Beth Vanhorn.
© 2018 John Wiley & Sons, Inc. Published 2018 by John Wiley & Sons, Inc.
Companion website: www.wiley.com/go/vanhorn/breeds

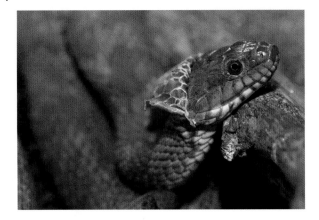

Figure 7.1 Ecdysis in a snake.

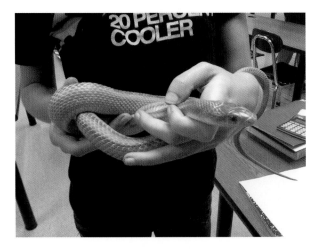

Figure 7.3 Snakes have no limbs and their bodies are covered in scales.

outside surface of their bodies, hence caution with handling and attention to proper sanitation are necessary. Reptiles cannot metabolize nutrients or synthesize vitamin D properly without ultraviolet (UV) lighting and suitable full-spectrum bulbs must be provided.

7.3 Types of Reptiles

7.3.1 Snakes

Snakes are one of the most recognizable classes of reptiles (Figure 7.3). There are over 2500 species of snakes in the world. The most commonly kept pet snakes are in the families of Boaidea, Pythonidae, and Colubridae. Boas originate from South and Central America and are constrictors, meaning that they capture and kill their prey by suffocation. Boas can grow to lengths of 18 feet or more and are popular pets owing to their wide color varieties and docile temperaments. Pythons are also constrictors and the most popular is the ball python, reaching lengths of around 5 feet. Other python species

may reach lengths of 20 feet or more and weigh over 200 pounds. Many also have unpredictable and less docile temperaments.

> ***Points to remember.*** There are more than 2500 species of snakes.

7.3.2 Lizards

Lizards come in a variety of sizes and colors (Figure 7.4). There are over 3500 species of lizards. Some lizards will grow to several inches in length and others can grow to over 10 feet. Lizards have four limbs and a long tail, both of which are quite strong. Many lizard species are native to the tropics or desert-like environments. Many lizards are docile but some can become nervous and quick and have a variety of temperaments, from some that never bite to those that are instinctively aggressive. Lizards have a thick, scaly skin that protects them from heat, sunlight, and dryness. They generally molt or shed their skin on an

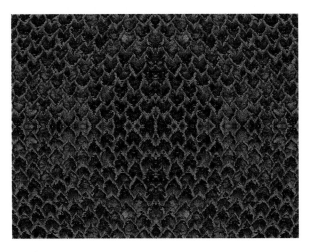

Figure 7.2 Scales on a lizard.

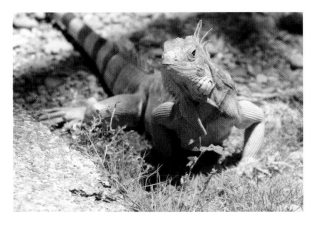

Figure 7.4 Lizards are covered in scutes and have four limbs.

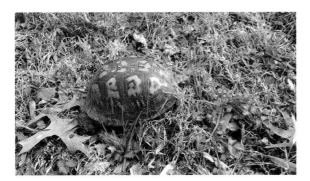

Figure 7.5 Box turtles are common pets.

ongoing basis. Some lizards are climbers and others live primarily on the ground. Lizards also include a group of reptiles called skinks, anoles, chameleons, geckos, iguanas, monitors, and dragons. Lizards are cold blooded and cannot regulate their own body heat internally and therefore require cages that have a supplemental heat source. Some types of lizards must maintain proper body temperatures in order to digest their food and utilize nutrients. Care must also be taken not to provide too hot a heat source that can lead to thermal burns or scalding.

> ***Points to remember.*** There are more than 3500 species of lizards.

7.3.3   Turtles

Turtles come in a variety of types based on their environment. There are over 290 species of turtles. They may be terrestrial or land living or they may be aquatic or semiaquatic species. Box turtles are the most commonly kept terrestrial species (Figure 7.5). Sliders, maps, and painted turtles are commonly kept aquatic species. Turtle shells may be hard or soft based on their environmental needs. In 1975, a US federal law banned the sale of turtles under 4 inches in length. Larger tortoise species may grow to sizes of over 3 feet wide and over 200 pounds in weight and can live for over 100 years.

Sources

American Reptile Association (ARA) (2016).
Society for the Study of Reptiles and Amphibians (SSAR) (2016).
APPA (2014) *2013–2014 APPA National Pet Owners Survey.* American Pet Product Association, Greenwich, CT.
AVMA (2012) *U.S. Pet Ownership & Demographics Sourcebook*, American Veterinary Medical Association, Schaumburg, IL.

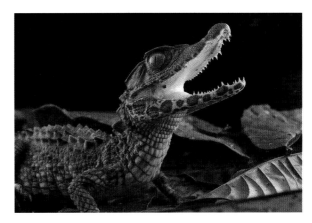

Figure 7.6 Caimans can grow to over 10 feet in length.

> ***Points to remember.*** There are more than 290 species of turtles.

7.3.4   Crocodiles and Alligators

There are around 23 different species of alligators and crocodiles. Crocodile and alligator species are not recommended as pets for beginner reptile owners. However, the most commonly kept species includes the caiman. Caimans are native to Central and South America (Figure 7.6). Caimans vary in size and, although shorter than alligators, they can still grow to over 10 feet in length. Many US states have laws regarding ownership of caimans and permits are required.

7.4   Summary

Reptiles vary in size, shape, temperament, and care needs. It is vital to research species prior to acquiring one as many reptiles have long life spans and require substantial maintenance and care. Reptiles have become a favorite companion pet and as there are many options regarding types of reptiles, there is a large demand for them.

Further Reading

Alderton, D. (ed.) (2014) *Practical Reptile Keeping*, Kelsey Publishing, Cudham.
Baby Professor (2015) *Reptiles of the World: Fun Facts for Kids*, CreateSpace.

8

Amphibian Species Identification

OBJECTIVES

Upon completion of this chapter, the reader should be able to:

- recognize common amphibian species;
- identify and describe Society for the Study of Amphibians and Reptiles (SSAR) recognized amphibian species;
- discuss and describe the types of amphibians.

8.1 Introduction

Amphibians include frogs, toads, salamanders, and newts. There are more than 4000 species of amphibians. Founded in 1958, the Society for the Study of Amphibians and Reptiles (SSAR) was established to advance research, conservation, and education concerning amphibians and reptiles. It is the largest international herpetological society, and is recognized worldwide for having the most diverse program of publications, meetings, and other activities. Amphibians, like reptiles, naturally harbor *Salmonella* bacteria and caution must be taken to sanitize hands properly after handling them. Also, some amphibian species are poisonous and these species are not recommended as pets.

Points to remember. There are more than 4000 species of amphibians.

8.2 Characteristics of Amphibians

Amphibians are all aquatic in nature, with some living primarily in water and others living on land or in combination. Amphibians do not like to be handled, making ownership more about observation, care, and providing a proper habitat or terrarium. Handling can also harm the

amphibian by introducing infection. Amphibians share the following characteristics:

- cold blooded/ectothermic;
- metamorphosis in life cycle;
- offspring live in water and have gills;
- adults develop lungs and breath through lungs and/or skin;
- may live in water, on land, or a combination;
- vertebrates;
- carnivores.

Frogs and toads are amphibians that do not have tails (Figure 8.1), a feature that differentiates them from salamanders and newts, which do have tails (Figure 8.2). Amphibians are cold-blooded animals that derive heat from outside their body. The body temperature of the amphibians depends on the outside surroundings. Hence the amphibians are very active in warm environments and become lethargic when exposed to low temperatures. As offspring amphibians begin their life cycle under water, breathing through gills. As they reach adulthood, they move to land and breathe with the help of either skin or lungs and develop legs. This metamorphosis occurs during the life of each amphibian.

8.3 Types of Amphibians

8.3.1 Frogs

Frogs are characterized by long hind legs, a short body, webbed toes, protruding eyes, and the absence of a tail (Figure 8.3). Most frogs have a semi-aquatic lifestyle, but move easily on land by jumping or climbing. The distribution of frogs ranges from tropic to subarctic regions, but most species are found in tropical rainforests. Consisting of more than 5000 species, they are among the most diverse groups of vertebrates. Some frog species are aquatic, living exclusively in the water. Others are terrestrial, living primarily on land, and some are arboreal and must have trees or limbs within their environment.

Veterinary Guide to Animal Breeds, First Edition. Beth Vanhorn.
© 2018 John Wiley & Sons, Inc. Published 2018 by John Wiley & Sons, Inc.
Companion website: www.wiley.com/go/vanhorn/breeds

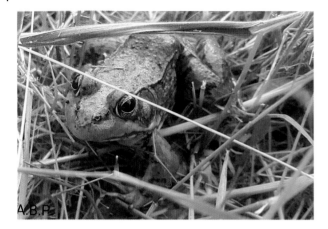

Figure 8.1 Example of a frog.

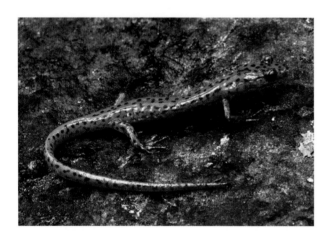

Figure 8.2 Example of a salamander.

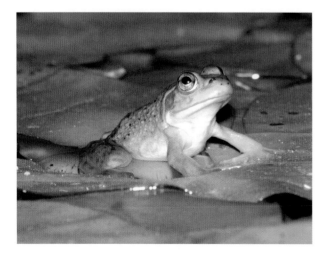

Figure 8.3 A bullfrog is a common pet.

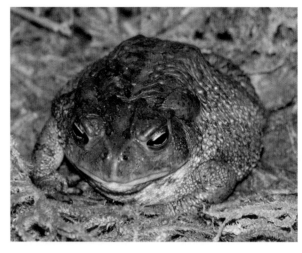

Figure 8.4 American toad.

> **Points to remember.** There are more than 5000 species of frogs.

8.3.2 Toads

Toads often have leathery skin for better water retention and a brown coloration for camouflage (Figure 8.4). They also tend to burrow. They are tailless and tend to be slightly larger in size than frogs. A distinction is often made between frogs and toads on the basis of their appearance, caused by the adaptation of toads to dry environments. Similarly to frogs, toads also go through a metamorphosis stage, from tadpole to adult.

8.3.3 Salamanders

Salamanders are the common name for approximately 500 species of amphibians. They are typically characterized by their slender bodies, short noses, and long tails (Figure 8.5). Most salamanders have four toes on their

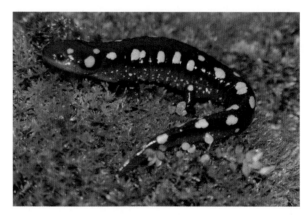

Figure 8.5 Spotted salamander.

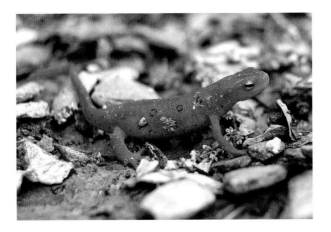

Figure 8.6 Red-spotted newt.

front legs and five on their rear legs. Their moist skin usually makes them reliant on habitats in or near water, or under some protection, such as a log, and often in a wetland. Some salamander species are fully aquatic throughout life, some take to the water occasionally, and some are entirely terrestrial as adults. Uniquely among vertebrates, they are capable of regenerating lost limbs, and also other body parts.

> ***Points to remember.*** There are more than 500 species of salamanders.

8.3.4 Newts

Newts are amphibians related to the salamander family, although not all aquatic salamanders are considered newts (Figure 8.6). Newts are found in North America, Europe, and Asia. Newts go through a metamorphosis in three distinct developmental life stages: aquatic larva, terrestrial juvenile or eft, and adult. Adult newts have lizard-like bodies and may be either fully aquatic or semi-aquatic, living terrestrially but returning to the water each year to breed. Newts, like salamanders, are also capable of regenerating lost limbs, and also other body parts.

8.4 Summary

Amphibians, like reptiles, can be kept as pets but it is helpful to research and have knowledge about the species of animal before purchasing one. Amphibians come in many shapes, sizes, and colors, and being able to identify and understand these animals will make owning one a much happier and safer experience.

Sources

Society for the Study of Amphibians and Reptiles (SSAR) (2016).
APPA (2014) *2013–2014 APPA National Pet Owners Survey.* American Pet Product Association, Greenwich, CT.
AVMA (2012) *U.S. Pet Ownership & Demographics Sourcebook*, American Veterinary Medical Association, Schaumburg, IL.

Further Reading

Howell, C.H. (2015) *National Geographic Pocket Guide to Reptiles and Amphibians of North America*, National Geographic, Washington, DC.
Mattison, C. (2013) *What Reptile? A Buyer's Guide for Reptiles and Amphibians*, Barron's Educational Series, Hauppauge, NY.

9

Cattle Breed Identification

Veterinary Guide to Animal Breeds, First Edition. Beth Vanhorn.
© 2018 John Wiley & Sons, Inc. Published 2018 by John Wiley & Sons, Inc.
Companion website: www.wiley.com/go/vanhorn/breeds

OBJECTIVES

Upon completion of this chapter, the reader should be able to:

- recognize common breeds of cattle species;
- identify and describe the National Cattlemen's Beef Association (NCBA) and the Purebred Dairy Cattle Association (PDCA) recognized cattle breeds;
- discuss and describe the two types of cattle.

9.1 Introduction

Cattle were first domesticated around 6500 BC. Cattle are raised in production systems for their meat, milk, and by-products. The United States Department of Agriculture (USDA) states that there are over 30 million beef cattle and 9 million dairy cattle in the world. The National Cattlemen's Beef Association (NCBA) was formed in 1898 and is one of the oldest and largest associations in the cattle industry: "This national trade association represents cattle producers, with more than 28,000 individual members and 64 state affiliate, breed, and industry organization members. Together NCBA represents more than 230,000 cattle breeders, producers, and feeders. NCBA works to advance the economic, political, and social interests of the US cattle business and to be an advocate for the cattle industry's policy positions and economic interests." The Purebred Dairy Cattle Association (PDCA) was founded in 1940 and is a "federation of the seven national dairy breed registry associations representing over 60,000 members. It provides leadership within the industry and conducts activities to increase the acceptance of purebred dairy cattle, while expanding opportunities for owners of dairy cattle to profit through improved management and marketing." There are over 900 different breeds of beef cattle but only seven recognized pure breeds of dairy cattle. Cross-breeding of cattle is common to produce further dual-purpose breeds that have the ability to provide both milk and meat.

Points to remember. There are more than 900 recognized cattle breeds.

9.2 Characteristics of Cattle

Cattle are bovines from the Bovidae family and domestic cattle are related to oxen, bison, and antelope. Cattle share the following characteristics:

- rectangular body shape;
- small heads;
- large, muscular bodies;
- herbivores;
- ruminants;
- eyes on side of head;
- cloven hooved;
- thick skin.

Cattle tend to be stocky, with long, rectangular bodies. Beef cattle are more muscular (Figure 9.1); dairy cattle have a truer rectangular shape with bony projections over the hind end (Figure 9.2). Some cattle breeds have a hump over the shoulder area. The head is small relative to body size, with a long, straight snout. Cattle have strong necks and prominent dewlaps located under the neck. Other physical characteristics vary between breed, such as the position of the ears or length of the legs and color and markings. Weight and height vary greatly between domestic cattle breeds. Some weigh more than 3000 pounds. Cattle are prey species. Their eyes are located on the sides of their heads, allowing them to capture movement around them, but they take longer to focus on specific objects. Their excellent peripheral vision creates a panorama effect on their sides. Their hearing tends to be sensitive to high-pitched noises, dairy breeds more so than beef breeds.

Cattle are herbivores and foragers and eat grass and hay sources, with a stomach system called ruminant that

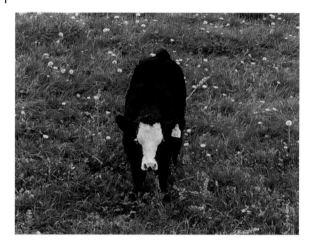

Figure 9.1 Example of a beef cow.

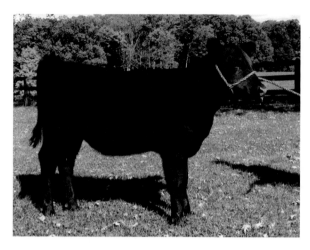

Figure 9.3 Black Angus beef cow.

has a stomach with four chambers for breaking down and digesting food. Cattle live an average of 15 years.

9.3 Types of Cattle

9.3.1 Beef Cattle

Beef cattle are raised for meat production and tend to be larger, more muscular, and more powerful in appearance (Figure 9.3). Beef cows are genetically bred to grow larger and faster. Many beef breeds have been modified genetically to adapt better to warm climates. Breeds of beef cattle are categorized by their geographical location of origin. American beef breeds were developed in the

United States from cow stock brought to the New World from other locations. American beef breeds include the Beefmaster, Brahman, Brangus, and Santa Gertrudis. British beef breeds are very numerous and commonly of moderate weight, well muscled, and have mild temperaments. British beef breeds include the Angus, Devon, Galloway, Hereford, Highland, and Shorthorn. Continental breeds are those that came to the United States from Western Europe between the 1960s and 1970s when many new breeds were introduced into the beef industry. These breeds include the Charolais, Chianina, Gelbvieh, Limousin, Maine-Anjou, Salers, and Simmental.

> **Points to remember.** Beef cattle are muscular and powerful in appearance.

9.3.2 Dairy Cattle

The dairy industry focus on a few breeds of cattle and many have been cross-bred to provide further by-products and dual-purpose production systems.

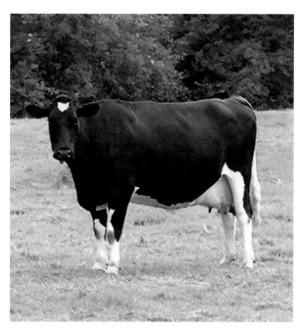

Figure 9.2 Example of a dairy cow.

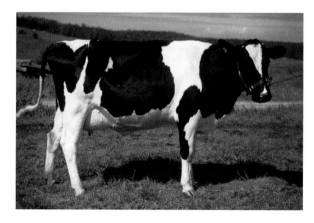

Figure 9.4 Holstein dairy cow.

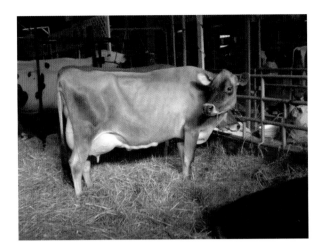

Figure 9.5 Jersey dairy cow.

Dairy breeds are often named for the area of origin and each breed has differences in the milk components produced. Breeds that produce milk higher in butterfat and proteins are often selected for milk sold for processing whereas other breeds are selected for milk volume (Figure 9.4). British dairy breeds include the Ayrshire, Guernsey, Jersey, and Milking Shorthorn (Figure 9.5).

Continental breeds include the Brown Swiss and the Holstein. Dairy cattle breeds have a body structure built for producing large quantities of milk. The hind quarters differ in that they have a more bony appearance and the bones of the pelvis are notable and appear to project upward and to the back in areas called the hooks and pins.

> **Points to remember.** Dairy cattle are angular and bony in shape.

9.4 Summary

The cattle industry is a large, multi-billion dollar industry with many countries leading in beef and dairy production. The beef industry generates over 20% of the total cash receipts in agriculture and the dairy industry over 11% of the total income generated in agriculture. Dairy cattle and beef cattle have identifiable differences and come in a variety of sizes, body conformations, and colors.

Sources

National Cattlemen's Beef Association (NCBA) (2016).
Purebred Dairy Cattle Association (PDCA) (2016).
United States Department of Agriculture (USDA) (2016).
USDA (2012) *2012 National Agricultural Statistics Service Survey*, United States Department of Agriculture, Washington, DC.

Further Reading

Byard, J. (2012) *Know Your Cows*, Fox Chapel Publishing, Petersburg, PA.
Lewis, C. (2014) *The Illustrated Guide to Cows*, Bloomsbury Publishing, London.
Purdy, H.R., Dawes, R.J., and Hough, R. (2008) *Breeds of Cattle*, 2nd edn., TRS Publishing, Springfield. MO.

10

Equine Breed Identification

OBJECTIVES

Upon completion of this chapter, the reader should be able to:

- recognize common breeds of equine species;
- identify and describe recognized equine breeds;
- discuss and describe the types of horses and equine species.

10.1 Introduction

Horses once served every role in a human's life, from food, to sources of travel and transportation, to a partner in recreation and physical therapy. Many horses still occupy traditional work roles in plowing and pulling wagons; however, most horses now serve recreational purposes. There are over 400 breeds of horses and each breed was developed for a specific use or task. Many breeds were developed in specific locations. Equine breeds include horses, donkeys, and mules. Donkeys and mules are a species rather than a breed. There are over 55 million horses in the world today, used for recreation, work, and racing and as therapy animals.

> **Points to remember.** There are more than 400 recognized horse breeds.

10.2 Characteristics of Equines

Equines come in a variety of heights and weights. Equines share the following characteristics:

- long, muscular neck;
- large bodied;
- erect ears;
- long mane/tail;
- long, lean legs;

- hooved;
- herbivores;
- non-ruminant.

Equines have four legs that are hooved. The hoof consists of a wall of horny keratin that grows down from a band called the coronet located at the top of the hoof (Figure 10.1). This process is similar to the way in which fingernails grow out from the cuticle. The sole of the horse foot is concave, with a fleshy wedge of tissue called the frog that projects forward from the heel. Inside the hoof is the coffin bone that takes the shape of the hoof. The sole and the frog protect the underside of the foot, while the fleshy tissues cushion each step like a spring. The long slim legs of the horse hold the large upper body and are common sites for lameness and injury.

The equine eyes are located on each side of the face, allowing vision of 300° in front and peripherally but not well to the rear. Horses have long, muscular necks with manes of hair that begin at the edge of the neck and grow out covering the side of the neck.

Equine species range in height from under 32 inches at the wither or shoulder area up to over 18 hands (1 hand equals 4 inches). Equines can weigh between 500 and over 1200 pounds. The average lifespan of the equine is between 20 and 25 years. Equines have four gaits or movements: the walk, the trot or jog, the canter or lope, and the gallop. All equine species may be trained to allow people to ride them, drive them under harness, or use them as pack animals. The equine is a versatile animal and may be trained to jump, navigate trail obstacles, work cattle, and many more disciplines. Adult horses have 40–42 teeth that develop for grinding food (Figure 10.2).

Horses may be classified by color, rather than breed. A "color" breed of horse is one known by its color pattern and is not a purebred horse since some color breeds, such as the Palomino and Buckskin, cannot be bred with each other and produce the same color 100% of the time (Figure 10.3). Common color breeds include the Buckskin, which has a golden shade body color with a black mane and tail and black leg markings. A Dun is a brownish red to golden color with the same shade or slightly

Veterinary Guide to Animal Breeds, First Edition. Beth Vanhorn.
© 2018 John Wiley & Sons, Inc. Published 2018 by John Wiley & Sons, Inc.
Companion website: www.wiley.com/go/vanhorn/breeds

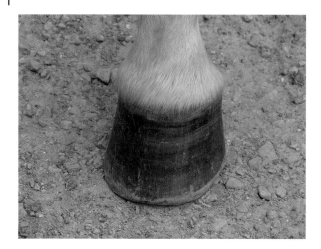

Figure 10.1 Horse hoof.

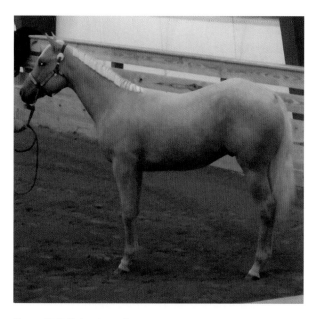

Figure 10.3 Palomino color.

darker shade of mane and tail and includes a cark stripe down the center of the back, called a dorsal stripe, and may have light stripes inside the legs, appearing like tiger stripe markings. A Palomino color is cream to golden with a white to silver mane and tail. A Pinto color is white with another darker color appearing in large patches over the body (Figure 10.4). A Roan color is a mixture of white hairs blended with red to black to produce a combination of shading from red to blue.

10.3 Types of Equines

10.3.1 Horses

Horses are the most common and populous of the equine species. Horses are divided into groups called ponies, light breeds, and draft breeds. Ponies are small equines less than 58 inches tall at the withers (Figure 10.5).

Each breed of pony has its set breed standard in height. Children are often the main enthusiasts of ponies, used for both riding and driving. Many ponies are too small for adults to ride. Common breeds of ponies include Shetland, Pony of the Americas (POA), and Welsh.

Light horses are those used primarily for riding and driving of light wagons or carriages. Light horses can be further defined into categories for which they were bred, such as stock types, warmbloods, and hunters. Stock type breeds have a muscular build desirable for working on a ranch or farm, such as the Quarter Horse (Figure 10.6). Warmbloods are a combination of draft size horses and light athletic horses that develop a large size and athletic body and substance. Hunter type horses are light, agile, and fast, with athletic abilities used in jumping obstacles (Figure 10.7). Light horse breeds include the Arabian, American Quarter Horse, American Paint

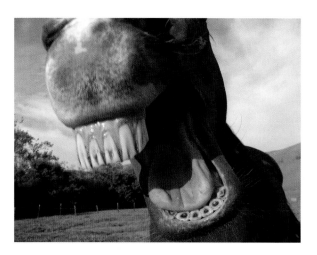

Figure 10.2 Horse teeth.

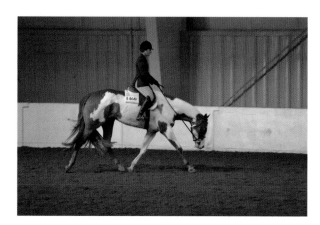

Figure 10.4 Pinto color. *Source*: Courtesy of Amanda Reed.

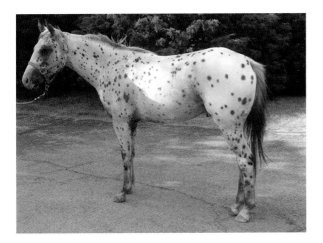

Figure 10.5 Pony of the Americas (POA).

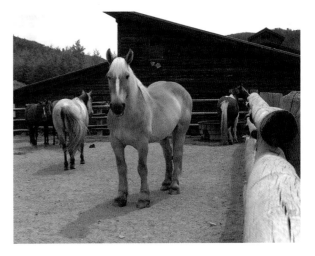

Figure 10.8 Belgian draft horse.

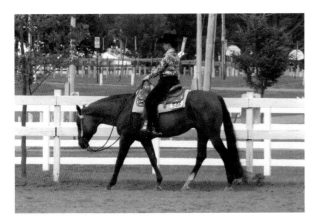

Figure 10.6 American Quarter Horse.

long distances (Figure 10.8). Draft horses are commonly used today in plowing of fields and pulling carriages and buggies in many religious sects. Draft horses are over 16 hands in height and may weigh over 2000 pounds. Common draft breeds include the Belgian, Clydesdale, Percheron, and Shire.

Miniature horses developed by breeding small horses with other small horses, many with Shetland pony blood (Figure 10.9). Despite being less than 34 inches at the withers, miniature horses, often called Minis, are not ponies. They must show the same characteristics, balance, and structure of a full size horse, in miniature form. They come in a variety of colors and color combinations.

10.3.2 Donkeys

Donkeys originated in Africa and were one of the first recorded equines used as work animals. Donkeys have large heads, large ears, and straight muscular necks (Figure 10.10). The tails are covered with short, bristled

Horse, Appaloosa, Morgan, Thoroughbred, Standardbred, and Tennessee Walking Horse.

Draft horses were developed for pulling heavy loads and were often crossed with lighter riding horses that had the endurance to pull smaller carriages full of people

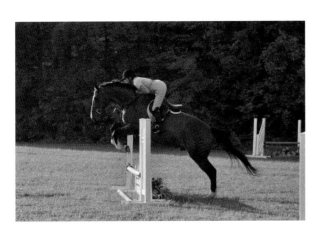

Figure 10.7 Hunter horse. *Source*: Courtesy of Amanda Reed.

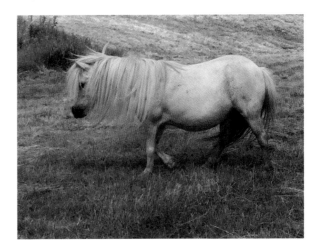

Figure 10.9 Miniature horse.

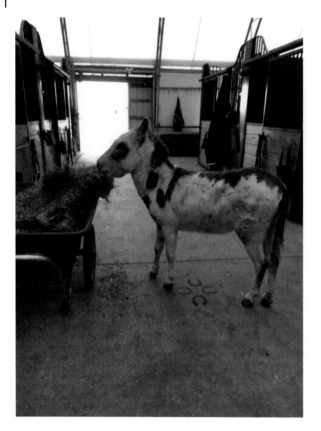

Figure 10.10 Donkey. *Source*: Courtesy of Jessica Berman.

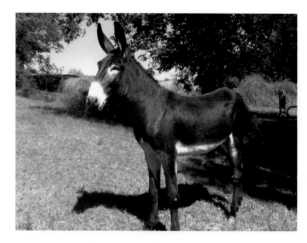

Figure 10.11 Mule.

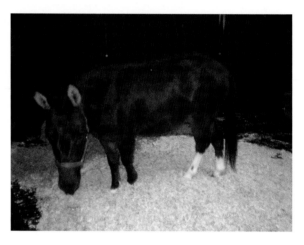

Figure 10.12 Miniature mule.

hair with the ends having a switch, much like a cow. Donkeys range in size from miniature to draft and are recognized by the American Donkey and Mule Society.

10.3.3 Mules

Mules are a result of crossing a female horse and a male donkey. A mule develops characteristics of both parents, with longer ears and a narrower body than those of a donkey (Figure 10.11). Mules are generally larger in size, with smooth hair and a tail like a horse. Both male and female mules are almost always sterile. A hinny results when a male horse is bred with a female donkey with the same characteristics as noted above. Mules can range in size from miniature to over 68 inches tall at the withers (Figure 10.12). Mules are also recognized by the American Donkey and Mule Society.

10.4 Summary

Equines developed based on location and type of use. Many horse breeds are found throughout the world. Horses have many colors, sizes, and characteristics based on their development and purpose. Equine species include horses, ponies, donkeys, and mules.

Sources

American Donkey and Mule Society (2016).
American Horse Council (2005) *American Horse Council Survey*, American Horse Council, Washington, DC.
USDA (2012) *2012 National Agricultural Statistics Service Survey*, United States Department of Agriculture, Washington, DC.

Further Reading

Draper, J. (2014) *The Complete Book of Horses*, Anness Publishing, London.
Ransford, S. (2010) *The Kingfisher Illustrated Horse and Pony Encyclopedia*, Kingfisher Publications, Boston, MA.
Walker, E. (2014) *The Horse*, Parragon Books, Bath.

11

Swine Breed Identification

OBJECTIVES

Upon completion of this chapter, the reader should be able to:

- recognize common breeds of pig species;
- identify and describe National Swine Registry (NSR) and the National Pork Producers Council (NPPC) recognized pig breeds;
- discuss and describe the two types of swine.

11.1 Introduction

Swine are known as pigs and hogs and were domesticated in 6500 BC. They have been a vital part of human life as a meat source, and are very efficient at converting food to meat. European explorers brought pigs to the New World and pigs were raised for their fat and lard production until the 1950s. More modern swine producers began to focus on raising animals as more lean and nutritious meat sources. This resulted in a high demand for pork and many breeds were developed for high-quality meat production. Today, many pigs that are raised for meat are cross-breeds. The National Swine Registry (NSR) was developed in 1994 to develop further the four major swine production breeds. The National Pork Producers Council was created to establish an organization that regulates consistent and responsible high-quality pork producers. Today, there are more than 62 million pigs raised in the United States alone.

11.2 Characteristics of Swine

Pigs are omnivores and will eat both meat- and plant-based food sources. Pigs come in a variety of sizes, weighing from 60 to over 300 pounds. Swine share the following characteristics:

- snout;
- erect or floppy ears;
- thick bodied;
- short neck;
- small eyes;
- long, pointed head;
- cloven hooved with four toes on each foot;
- large canine teeth protruding from the mouth;
- tufts of hair;
- cork-screw tails.

Pigs are intelligent and social animals and are generally also clean animals (Figure 11.1). They are near-sighted and use their sense of hearing and smell to guide them in specific directions. Their highly sensitive and characteristically shaped snout is used to sniff and burrow. Sweat glands are located only on the snout and this is one reason why they love to dig and burrow in mud. Pigs can be quite independent animals. They are characterized by their backfat, which is the thickness of fat located along the back and sides of the pig (Figure 11.2).

11.3 Types of Swine

Swine types are based on the meat sources that are suited for production systems and body types. Pork is a versatile meat that is lean and produces bacon, lard, ham, loin, and chops. Bacon-type hogs are the longer body type breeds with large body size and were developed to produce large amounts of bacon from the sides of the pig (Figure 11.3). Ham-type breeds are lean in meat and tend to be medium sized with well-developed muscling over the hind end quarters (Figure 11.4). Ham meat sources include the rump and hind leg of the pig, which can be divided into the butt half (rump) and the shank half (leg).

Veterinary Guide to Animal Breeds, First Edition. Beth Vanhorn.
© 2018 John Wiley & Sons, Inc. Published 2018 by John Wiley & Sons, Inc.
Companion website: www.wiley.com/go/vanhorn/breeds

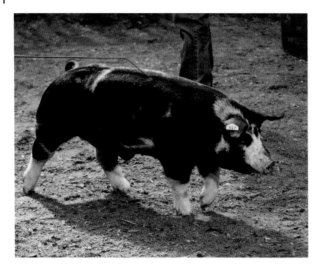

Figure 11.1 Pigs are intelligent and easily trained to be shown. *Source*: Courtesy of Wendy MacDonald.

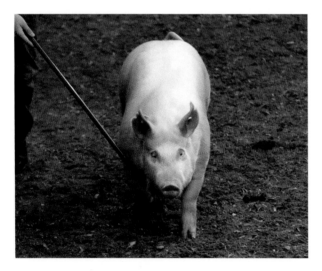

Figure 11.2 Example of backfat on a pig showing the thickness of fat along the back. *Source*: Courtesy of Wendy MacDonald.

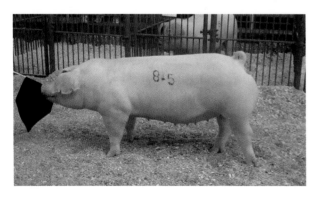

Figure 11.3 A bacon-type pig breed, the American Landrace.

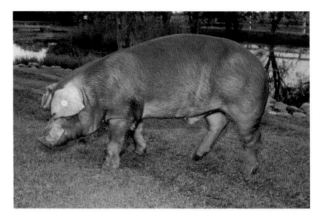

Figure 11.4 A ham-type pig breed, the Duroc.

The loin area is also a heavily muscled area located over the shoulder to the hind limbs along both sides of the backbone. These cuts of meat include the ribs, sirloin, pork chops, and center cut.

11.4 Breeds of Swine

Most pigs are bred by cross-breeding for specific traits of contributing breeds. Some crosses focus on producing maternal traits that contribute to success and efficiency in raising offspring. Other crosses focus on production traits that contribute to high-quality meat and uniform and marketable carcass. Uniformity of the carcass is highly important in the US pork industry. Many purebreed swine have been developed for specific traits that are now used both in pure breeding and in cross-breeding production systems. There are more than 20 recognized pure breeds and more than 50 cross-breeds.

> **Points to remember.** There are more than 20 recognized pure swine breeds and more than 50 cross-breeds.

11.4.1 American Breeds

American breeds include the Chester White, Duroc, Hereford, Poland China, and Spots. The Chester White originated in Pennsylvania and is a moderate-sized white hog with forward-flopping ears (Figure 11.5). The Duroc was developed in the eastern United States in the mid-1800s and is a distinctive red breed ranging from light red to mahogany red in color. The ears flop slightly forward and this popular breed of pig grows quickly. The Hereford was developed in the mid-western United States and is marked similar to the cattle breed with a red body and white face and legs (Figure 11.6). Herefords are known

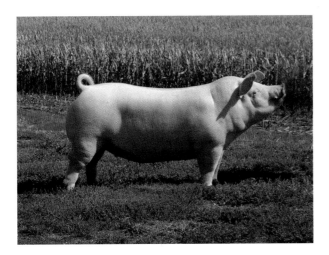

Figure 11.5 Chester White.

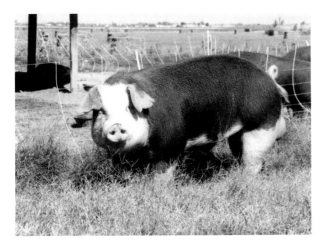

Figure 11.6 Hereford.

to be good mothers that have large litter numbers. The Poland China breed originated in Ohio in the early 1800s and is large with a black body with white face, feet and tail (Figure 11.7). These pigs have forward-flopping ears and are known to produce low backfat and large loins. The

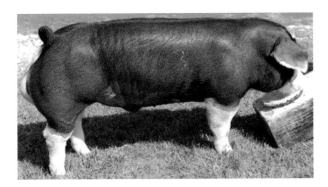

Figure 11.7 Poland China.

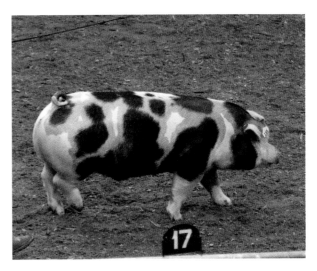

Figure 11.8 Spots. *Source*: Courtesy of Wendy MacDonald.

Spots breed was developed in Indiana and is large bodied with black and white spotted patterns (Figure 11.8).

11.4.2 British Breeds

British breeds include the Berkshire, Hampshire, and Tamworth. The Berkshire was developed in the eighteenth century in the Berkshire region of England (Figure 11.9). The pigs are black with white feet, faces, and tails. Ears stand erect. The Hampshire was developed in the Hampshire region of England and is black and white in color with the white pattern forming a belt around the front quarter and including the front legs (Figure 11.10). The pigs have erect ears and have desirable lean meat. The Tamworth originated in Ireland and England in the nineteenth century and is one of the oldest pure breeds of swine (Figure 11.11). The animals are red in color with erect ears and long faces and a very rounded back. The females have good maternal qualities

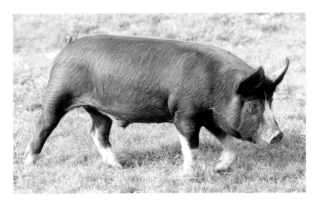

Figure 11.9 Berkshire.

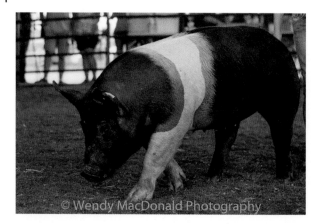

Figure 11.10 Hampshire. *Source*: Courtesy of Wendy MacDonald.

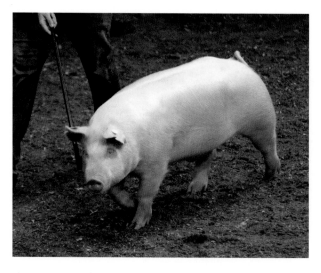

Figure 11.12 Landrace. *Source*: Courtesy of Wendy MacDonald.

and produce large litters. They are especially known as a high-quality bacon-producing meat breed.

11.4.3 European Breeds

European breeds include the Landrace, Pietrain, and Yorkshire. The Landrace is a large breed white hog that originated in Denmark (Figure 11.12). They are known for producing large litters and the females have good maternal traits. Landrace pigs have lean bodies that are relatively long with ears that flop over the eyes and face. Pietrains were developed in Belgium in the 1950s and are a medium sized breed with black and white spots and erect ears (Figure 11.13). They have well-muscled hams and do not have good maternal qualities or good milk production. The Yorkshire was developed in the Yorkshire region of England and imported into the United States in the 1800s. Similarly to the Landrace, these pigs are a large breed with a long white body and erect ears (Figure 11.14). They grow fast and use their feed efficiently.

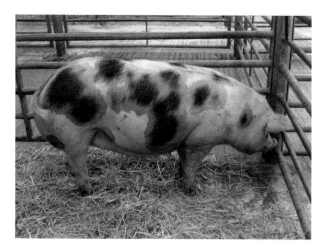

Figure 11.13 Pietrain.

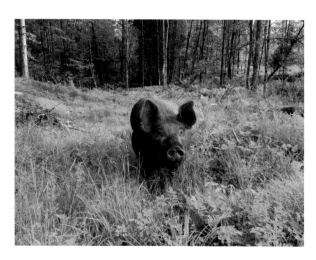

Figure 11.11 Tamworth.

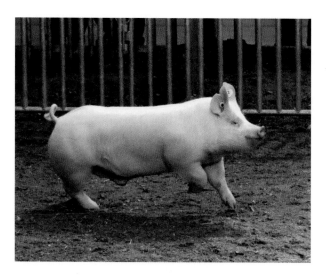

Figure 11.14 Yorkshire. *Source*: Courtesy of Wendy MacDonald.

11.4.4 Asian Breeds

Several Asian breeds have begun to become popular as swine breeds as they grow quickly, have large litters, and reach puberty fairly quickly. Their growth is slower than that of the other traditional breeds, so their use has been limited.

11.5 Summary

The swine industry in a large agricultural industry in the United States economyl. Many breeds have been developed with specific traits in mind to help improve the quality of meat and the production systems. Leanness in meat quality continues to be a priority for swine producers in response to consumers wanting to eat a healthier product, and the National Pork Producers Council is committed to setting standards to do that. Many breeds have been developed via cross-breeding and crossing of breeds is still useful today to improve the commercial industry.

Sources

National Pork Producers Council (2016).
National Swine Registry (NSR) (2016).
USDA (2012) *2012 National Agricultural Statistics Service Survey*, United States Department of Agriculture, Washington, DC.

Further Reading

Byard, J. (2012) *Know Your Pigs*, Fox Chapel Publishing, Petersburg, PA.
Lewis, C. (2001) *The Illustrated Guide to Pigs*, Bloomsbury Publishing, London.

12

Sheep Breed Identification

12.1 Introduction

Sheep were among the first production animals to be domesticated. In the 1800s the focus of sheep production was primarily on wool. Today, sheep are raised for wool, meat, and hobby. The American Sheep Industry Association (ASI) was founded in 1865. The goal of the ASI is to promote and develop further the well-being of the sheep industry with regard to wool, meat, and lamb production and to educate and improve the health of sheep. There are more than 200 different breeds of purebred sheep and many production systems allow cross-breeding to produce specific qualities. There are over one billion sheep raised in the world today.

Points to remember. There are more than 200 recognized sheep breeds.

12.2 Characteristics of Sheep

Sheep can easily be confused with some goat breeds. Sheep range in weight from 100 to 350 pounds. Sheep share the following characteristics:

- thick wool coat;
- polled or horned;
- upper lip with ruminant division;
- herbivores;
- docked tail;
- erect or floppy ears.

A sheep typically has a docked tail that lies flat for wool sanitation and health reasons (Figure 12.1). Sheep may have ears that stand erect or may be floppy. Sheep hair is typically wool and may be fine, medium or long. Wool quality may also be described by texture. Owing to the wool length and texture, most sheep require regular shearing. Many sheep breeds are polled and if horns do develop they tend to curl in loops at the side of the head. Sheep are grazers and tend to forage on short grass that is tender. Sheep are naturally flock animals that tend to be distant and aloof with humans.

12.3 Classes of Sheep

12.3.1 Wool Breeds

Sheep are classified based on the type of wool they produce. Fine wool sheep are bred primarily to produce wool for clothing, textiles, and synthetic fabrics. Fine wool sheep include the Merino and Rambouillet (Figure 12.2). Medium wool breeds are used primarily for meat production and have a medium length wool coat. Medium wool breeds include the Cheviot, Dorset, Hampshire, Oxford, and Suffolk (Figure 12.3). Long wool sheep breeds were originally developed in England and have coarse wool and poor-quality carcasses. They are popular in cross-breeding systems and are less popular in the United States. Long wool breeds include the Cotswold and Lincoln. Cross-bred wool types of sheep were developed to produce a good-quality meat breed and high-production wool breed. They have also been bred to have strong flocking instincts. Cross-bred wool breeds include the Columbia and Corriedale (Figure 12.4).

12.3.2 Hair Breeds

Hair sheep breeds have become more popular in the sheep industry. The hair breeds develop more hair

Veterinary Guide to Animal Breeds, First Edition. Beth Vanhorn.
© 2018 John Wiley & Sons, Inc. Published 2018 by John Wiley & Sons, Inc.
Companion website: www.wiley.com/go/vanhorn/breeds

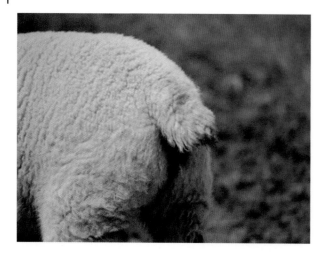

Figure 12.1 Sheep with docked tail.

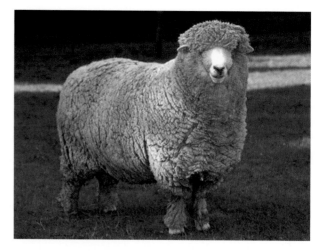

Figure 12.4 Corriedale.

follicles than wool follicles. Hair breeds do not require shearing as their hair sheds naturally. Most hair sheep breeds were developed in tropical regions and do well in warmer climates and are resistant to many diseases. Hair sheep breeds include the Katahdin, Barbados, and St. Croix (Figure 12.5).

> ***Points to remember.*** Hair sheep breeds do not require shearing as their hair sheds naturally.

12.3.3 Other Breeds

Other wool types include carpet breeds, in which the wool is coarse and long, and these are best suited for non-clothing products. Fur sheep are bred specifically for the pelt, which is typically harvested from lambs at a few days of age and used primarily for coats and other heavy apparel.

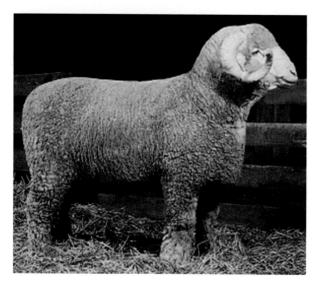

Figure 12.2 Rambouillet.

Figure 12.3 Suffolk.

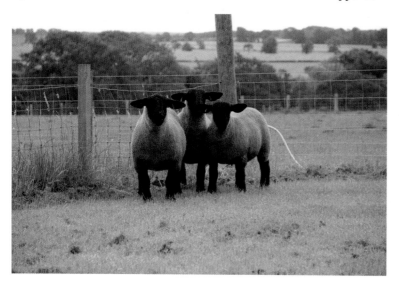

Figure 12.5 Katahdin.

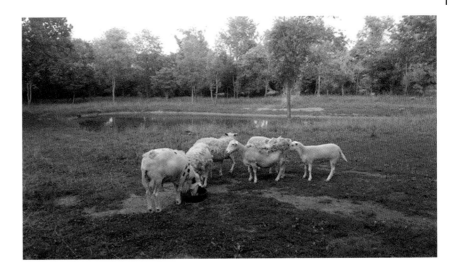

12.4 Breeds of Sheep

12.4.1 Fine Wool Breeds

Fine wool breeds of sheep include the white Debouillet, which thrives best in the western rangelands. They are solid white and medium sized. The Merino is a classic Spanish breed that has varying wrinkles over the skin and develops a fine fleece hair coat that is white in color (Figure 12.6). It is a medium-sized breed and one of the oldest sheep breeds, and it produces high-quality wool. The Rambouillet was developed in France and is a large breed with a meaty carcass, and is white in color, with fleece developing over the entire body except the face.

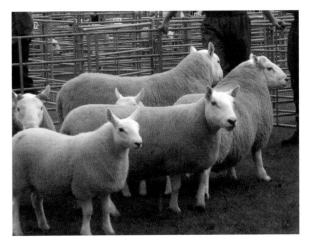

Figure 12.7 Cheviot.

12.4.2 Medium Wool Breeds

Medium wool breeds include the Cheviot, a small, white sheep developed in England that is distinctive in that it has black feet, a stocky build, and moderate fleece over the body except with no wool growing on the legs or head (Figure 12.7). The Dorset is a medium-sized white sheep that was developed in England (Figure 12.8). These sheep may be horned or polled and are white in color, and are multi-production breeds used for meat, wool, and milk.

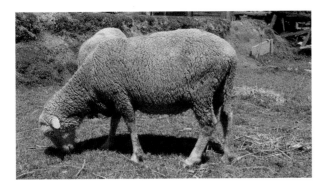

Figure 12.6 Merino.

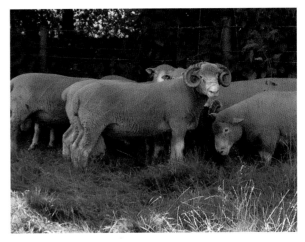

Figure 12.8 Dorset.

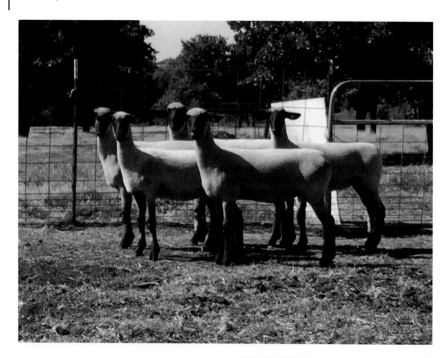

Figure 12.9 Hampshire.

The Finnish Landrace is a light-bodied white sheep from Finland and are most commonly used in cross-breeding programs. The Hampshire is a medium-sized sheep with a white body and black over the legs, face, and ears. Some wool is found over the face but may not come down to eye level (Figure 12.9). These sheep may have some wool on the lower legs but large amounts are discouraged. They are naturally polled with stocky builds.

The Montadale is a medium-sized to large breed that is solid white with no wool over the face and legs. The sheep are naturally polled and are dual purpose for wool and meat. The Oxford is a large breed developed in England with gray to brown color over the legs face, ears, and nose and a white body (Figure 12.10). Wool grows on the face and between the eyes. The Shropshire is a hardy breed that is small in size, polled, and has a dark face and legs and wool over the face. Southdowns are grayish brown in color with wool developing over the entire body and are naturally polled (Figure 12.11). The Suffolk is the most popular sheep breed in the United States and is a large muscular breed with a white body and black on the legs, head, and ears. These sheep are polled, with no wool development on the legs. The Tunis was developed in Africa and is a medium-sized breed with coarse wool and an angular frame (Figure 12.12), and with reddish hair on the face and lower legs.

12.4.3 Long Wool Breeds

Long wool breeds include the Cotswold, which is an English breed that is polled and has a long curling wool coat that hangs in locks between 8 and 10 inches in length. The sheep are primarily white but may have dark

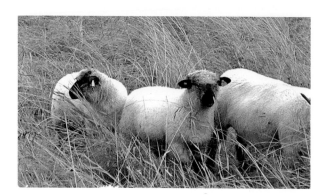

Figure 12.10 Oxford.

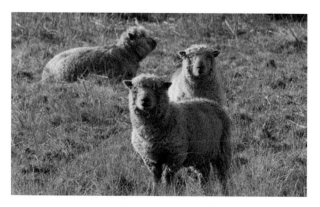

Figure 12.11 Southdown.

Figure 12.12 Tunis.

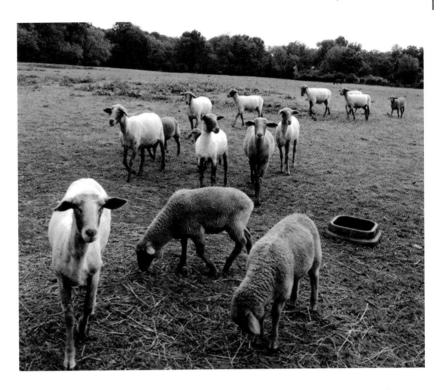

spots on the legs. The Lincoln is the largest sheep breed and may weigh over 350 pounds (Figure 12.13). These sheep are white with white faces and legs and are polled. They develop long fleece locks that can grow to 15 inches in length. The Romney is a large white breed developed in England as a dual-purpose breed. It has the finest fleece of the long wool breeds and the wool is commonly used for hand spinning.

12.4.4 Cross-Bred Wool Breeds

The cross-bred wool types include the popular Columbia, which was developed in the United States as a large breed with a lean build (Figure 12.14). These sheep are white in color with wool developing on the body but not over the head and face. The Corriedale is a white to gray color sheep developed in New Zealand. The Targhee

is a newer breed that was developed in the United States and is a medium-sized to large white sheep.

12.4.5 Hair Breeds

The hair sheep breeds are becoming more popular. The Barbados Blackbelly sheep are uniform with brown hair over the body and black hair on the legs, nose, forehead, and ears (Figure 12.15). Males have longer hair under the neck and over the brisket. The breed is polled and has heavily muscling over the hindquarters. The Dorper was developed in South Africa and is a mutton-type hair breed, raised for both meat and hair. These sheep have

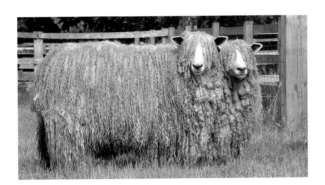

Figure 12.13 Lincoln.

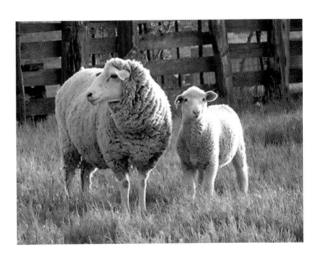

Figure 12.14 Columbia.

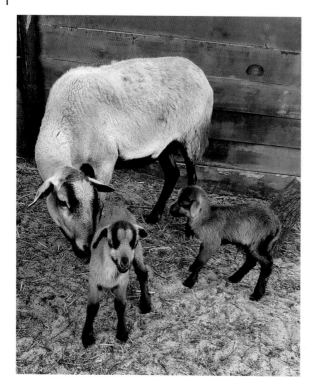

Figure 12.15 Barbados Blackbelly.

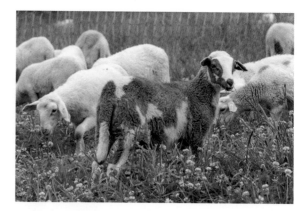

Figure 12.16 St. Croix.

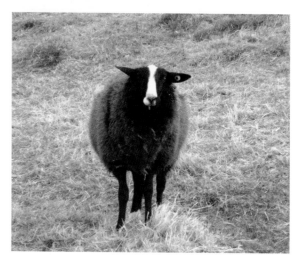

Figure 12.17 Black-faced Highland.

white bodies and most have a black head, although some may have a white head. The breed is hardy and grows quickly. The Katahdin is the most popular hair breed to be developed in the United States. These sheep are hardy animals that produce high-quality meat carcasses. They can be any color and typically have a double coat that consists of coarse outer hair fibers and an undercoat of fine wool fibers. The undercoat sheds naturally. The St. Croix was developed in the Virgin Islands and is adaptable to many climate types (Figure 12.16). The sheep are solid white and, depending on climate, may develop a thicker hair coat in cooler areas.

12.4.6 Carpet Breeds

The carpet wool breed is an old Scottish breed known as the Black-faced Highland, which is small in size with a white body and black face and legs, and has a long, coarse wool coat with curling horns (Figure 12.17). The fur sheep breed is the Karakul breed raised for its pelt and developed in Asia.

12.5 Summary

The sheep industry has contracted over the years but remains popular for the production of wool and meat. Consumer demand has decreased but the popularity of hobby farms has been increasing. Sheep are classified by their wool types, and knowledge and identification of breeds are based on the length and type of hair or wool that is produced.

Sources

American Sheep Industry Association (ASI) (2016).
USDA (2012) *2012 National Agricultural Statistics Service Survey*, United States Department of Agriculture, Washington, DC.

Further Reading

Parkin, S.R. (2013) *British Sheep Breeds*, Shire Publications, London.
Robson, D. and Ekarius, C. (2013) *The Field Guide to Fleece: 100 Sheep Breeds and How to Use Their Fibers*, Storey Publishing, North Adams, MA.

13

Goat Breed Identification

OBJECTIVES

Upon completion of this chapter, the reader should be able to:

- recognize common breeds of goat species;
- identify and describe American Goat Society (AGS) and American Dairy Goat Association (ADGA) recognized goat breeds;
- discuss and describe the classes of goats.

13.1 Introduction

Goats were domesticated around the same time as sheep and are also one of the oldest domesticated types of production animals. Goats serve as a multi-purpose animal in that they may be used for their hair, pelt, milk and meat. The market for goats has been low but meat production has been increasing over the years. The American Dairy Goat Association (ADGA) was founded in 1904 to collect, preserve, and record the pedigrees of dairy goat breeds and provide services and management to dairy goat breeders. The American Goat Society (AGS) originated in 1935 as a way to develop dairy goat breeds further. Today, it recognizes all pure- and cross-bred goat breeds. Currently there are more than 590 million goats raised in the world, and there are over 300 different types of goat breeds.

> **Points to remember.** There are more than 300 recognized breeds of goats.

13.2 Characteristics of Goats

Goats can easily be confused for sheep, especially those that have a longer hair coat that resembles that of wool. Goats have different hair types, from short to long and luxurious in texture, and range in weight from 20 to 250 pounds. Goats share the following characteristics:

- hair or fleece coat;
- horns;
- beards;
- large eyes with rectangular pupils;
- ruminants;
- herbivores;
- long tails.

Goats typically have erect or floppy ears and some breeds have no external ear flaps. Goat tails are typically held up high in the air. Goats are usually naturally horned, with more narrow, upright, and less curved horns than in sheep. Male goats tend to have a distinctly strong odor during the mating season. Goats have a naturally curious demeanor and are relatively independent. Goats like to rear up on their hind limbs and butt with their heads. Goats are grazers that will naturally browse, preferring to eat leaves, twigs, vines, and shrubs. They are very agile and will stand on their hind legs to reach vegetation. Goats like to eat the tops of plants.

13.3 Classes of Goats

13.3.1 Meat Goats

Goats are classified by their production type: meat, hair and dairy. Meat breed goats are raised for their meat, hide and pelts. They are highly meat productive and have-quality meat carcass characteristics. Some goats produce good-quality meat (called chevon), such as the Boer and Spanish breeds (Figure 13.1). Meat goats also are highly selected for their hides and pelts. Dairy goat breeds are raised for milk production (Figure 13.2). Many dairy goat breeds may also serve as dual purpose for their hair or meat. Dairy products include butter made from the cream of goat's milk, soft and hard cheeses, and fresh and evaporated milk, which tends to be more palatable than cow's milk and is much healthier for those with lactose intolerance.

Veterinary Guide to Animal Breeds, First Edition. Beth Vanhorn.
© 2018 John Wiley & Sons, Inc. Published 2018 by John Wiley & Sons, Inc.
Companion website: www.wiley.com/go/vanhorn/breeds

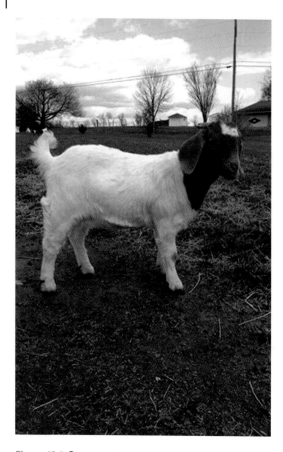

Figure 13.1 Boer meat goat.

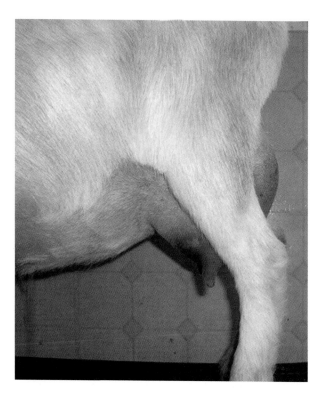

Figure 13.2 Dairy goat udder.

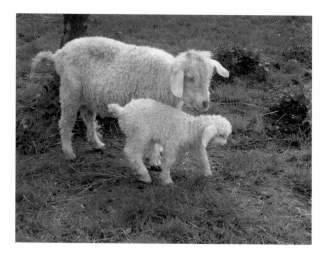

Figure 13.3 Angora goat.

13.3.2 Hair Breeds

Hair products from goats are primarily mohair and cashmere, which are fine hair harvested to make clothing, fabric, and other fiber by-products. Mohair is typically harvested from the Angora goat; cashmere is the fine undercoat of goats and can be harvested from any goat (Figure 13.3). Mohair and cashmere from solid-colored breeds are the most popular.

13.4 Breeds of Goats

Common goat breeds include the Angora, which was developed in Asia specifically for the production of mohair. Angora goats are white and have a fleece hair coat that grows long on the body, with no hair growth over the face. Most Angora goats develop horns and may serve as a dual-purpose animal for meat production. The Boer goat is the most popular meat-type goat breed and was developed in South America (Figure 13.4). These goats have a short, white hair coat with a variety of red markings. They may be horned or polled. The Alpine was developed in France as a dairy goat breed and has a variety of colors ranging through red, fawn, black and white or patterned with white (Figure 13.5). They have a short, fine hair coat with longer hair growth down the center of the back. The ears stand erect. The LaMancha goat is one of the more easily identifiable goat breeds (Figure 13.6). It has extremely short external ear flaps ranging from a gopher ear with no ear flap up to 1 inch in length or an elf ear up to 2 inches in length. This is primarily a dairy goat breed that can be any color or combination of colors.

The Nubian goat, developed in Africa, is a high-producing dairy goat breed with a high butterfat content in the milk (Figure 13.7). The Nubian can be any

Figure 13.4 Boer goats.

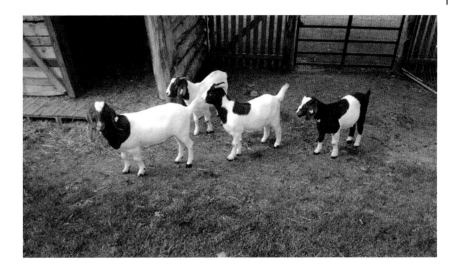

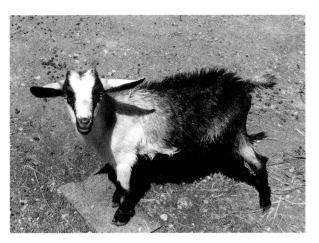

Figure 13.5 Alpine goat.

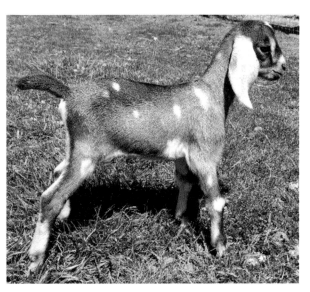

Figure 13.7 Nubian goat.

color or combination of colors but is recognized by its long, droopy ears and a Roman-shaped nose profile. Pygmy goats are popular as pets owing to their small size (Figure 13.8). They were developed in Africa and imported to zoos and petting zoos. They are less than 23 inches in height, with short legs and long bodies, and

come in a variety of colors and color combinations. They may be used for milk and meat but are most commonly seen as pets. The Saanen goat is cream to white in color and was developed in Switzerland (Figure 13.9). Most are

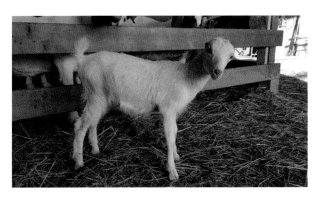

Figure 13.6 LaMancha goat.

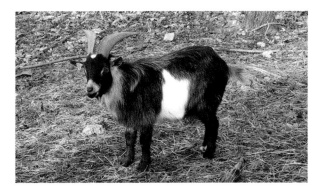

Figure 13.8 Pygmy goat.

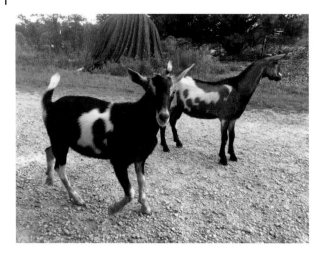

Figure 13.9 Saanen goat.

polled, with erect ears, and they often have beards. Spanish goats are raised primarily for meat but can serve a dual purpose for milk. They come in a variety of color combinations and have long, curved horns, pronounced hair over the eyes and face, and a long beard. The Toggenburg goat was developed in Switzerland and is fawn to dark brown in color, with a distinctive white line from the eyes down to the muzzle. They have erect ears and may be horned or polled. Some may develop a wattle of skin located beneath the chin.

13.5 Summary

Goat production has been on the increase in the United States with milk, meat, and pet popularity. Mohair tends to be the most popular fiber produced by goats. Knowledge of common goat breeds and their uses will help identify the breeds better.

Sources

American Dairy Goat Association (ADGA) (2016).
American Goat Society (AGS) (2016).
USDA (2012) *2012 National Agricultural Statistics Service Survey*, United States Department of Agriculture, Washington, DC.

Further Reading

Bahr, H. (2015) *Goats: Wild and Domestic Breeds Around the World*, CreateSpace.

14

Poultry Breed Identification

OBJECTIVES

Upon completion of this chapter, the reader should be able to:

- recognize common breeds of poultry species;
- identify and describe American Poultry Association (APA) recognized poultry breeds;
- discuss and describe the classes of poultry.

14.1 Introduction

Poultry is a broad term that classifies birds used in production systems and includes chickens, ducks, turkeys, geese, and ratites. The American Poultry Association (APA) was founded in 1873 to oversee and standardize the exhibition of poultry. Today, its mission is to protect, promote and preserve the standard-bred poultry industry in all of its phases. The APA was the first developed livestock association in the United States. There are more than 200 breeds of chickens recognized today. Turkeys are classified as one breed with over 18 varieties. There are over 100 domesticated duck and goose breeds. Many poultry species have become popular to raise for production and as pets and hobbies.

> **Points to remember.** There are more than 200 recognized chicken breeds.

14.2 Characteristics of Poultry

14.2.1 Chickens

Chickens are classified as the most common type of poultry raised for production. They are raised for meat, eggs, feathers and by-products. Chickens share the following characteristics:

- feathers;
- two wings;
- two limbs;
- beak;
- comb.

Chickens come in a variety of sizes and colors and their most distinguishing characteristic is that they are covered in feathers (Figure 14.1). Chickens have a beak, a fleshy comb growth located on the top of the head, two wings, and two limbs, and are rather social animals.

14.2.2 Turkeys

Turkeys are larger than chickens and have a large body covered in feathers (Figure 14.2). They are the only domestic poultry species of North American origin. Many developed from wild turkeys.

14.2.3 Waterfowl

Waterfowl are birds that spend the majority of their time on the water. Ducks and geese are included in this category. Ducks are smaller than geese (Figure 14.3). Geese are the largest of the domestic waterfowl and both ducks and geese are raised for meat, feathers, and down and as pets (Figure 14.4). Geese tend to be territorial and can become aggressive when someone enters their space.

14.3 Classes of Poultry

14.3.1 Chickens

Chickens are divided into different classes, breeds, and varieties. Class indicates the region of origin, breed indicates a set of birds with similar characteristics, and variety indicates a subgroup within a breed based on color and markings. Feather pattern and comb type are examples of features that may identify different varieties within a breed (Figure 14.5). *The American Standard of*

Veterinary Guide to Animal Breeds, First Edition. Beth Vanhorn.
© 2018 John Wiley & Sons, Inc. Published 2018 by John Wiley & Sons, Inc.
Companion website: www.wiley.com/go/vanhorn/breeds

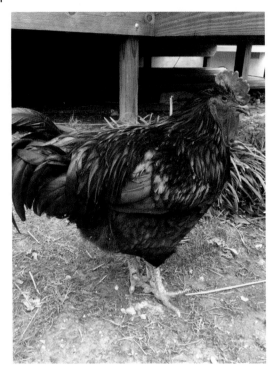

Figure 14.1 Chicken.

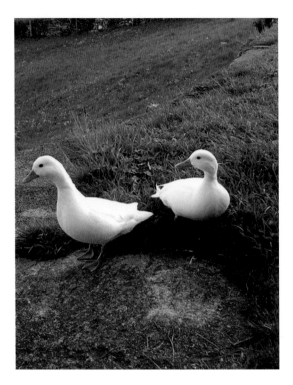

Figure 14.3 Ducks.

Perfection has been a publication of the APA since 1874 and describes the characteristics of each class and breed of chicken in the United States. Most standard breeds are moderate to large in size.

The American Class includes chicken breeds developed primarily in the Americas. The Asiatic Class includes breeds developed in Asia. The English Class includes breeds developed in Great Britain and the British Empire. The Mediterranean Class are breeds developed in countries found around the Mediterranean Sea. The Continental Class developed on the European continent.

14.3.2 Ducks and Geese

Duck breeds are determined by weight and size. The heavyweight birds range from 10 to 12 pounds for adult drakes and from 7 to 9 pounds for ducks. Medium-weight

Figure 14.2 Turkeys.

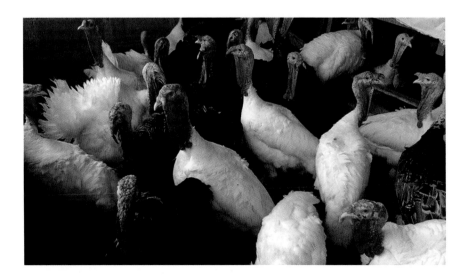

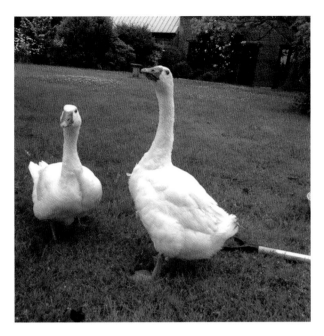

Figure 14.4 Geese.

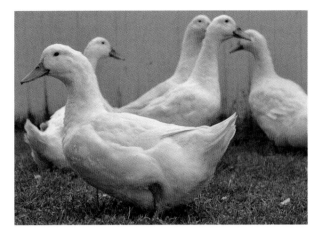

Figure 14.6 Pekin ducks.

birds range from 7 to 8 pounds for adult drakes and from 6 to 7 pounds for ducks (Figure 14.6). Lightweight birds weigh between 4 and 5 pounds for adult drakes and ducks. Geese are classified similarly to ducks, with heavy-weight, medium-weight and lightweight categories (Figure 14.7).

14.3.3 Ratites

The ratites are large birds raised for production, but owing to their large size they are not capable of flight. Ratites include the ostrich, rhea, and emu. Other common types of poultry raised for production purposes include guinea fowl, peafowl, pigeons, and quail (Figure 14.8). All of these birds are raised for meat, feathers, hides, oils, and other by-products.

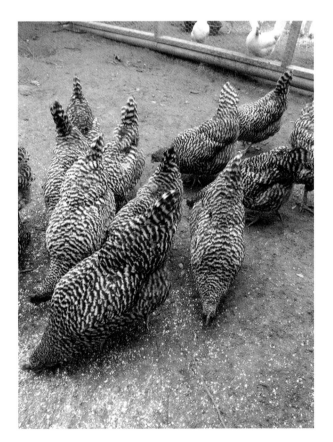

Figure 14.5 Plymouth Rock.

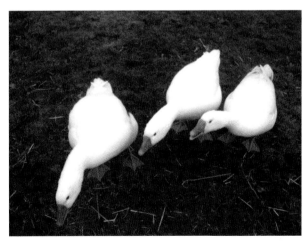

Figure 14.7 Embden geese.

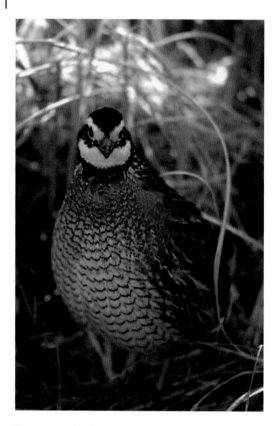

Figure 14.8 Quail.

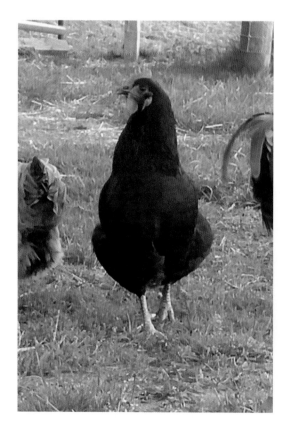

Figure 14.9 Ameraucana.

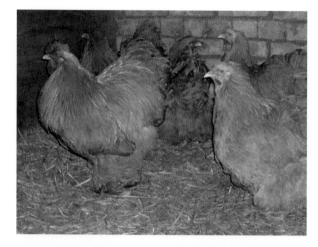

Figure 14.10 Cochin.

14.4 Breeds of Poultry

14.4.1 Chicken Breeds

Chicken breeds are considered production birds in the United States and are of standard breeds as defined by the APA *Standard of Perfection*. Most of the bantam breeds have been developed from miniaturization of a standard breed. The Ameraucana chicken is a dual-purpose breed in many color varieties that lays blue-colored eggs (Figure 14.9). They are a miscellaneous breed recognized by the APA and do not fit in any of the standard categories. The Araucana is a South American breed known commonly as the "Easter Egg Chicken" because of its variety of blue-colored shells. It is also a dual-purpose breed and was the foundation of the Ameraucana. The Ancona is

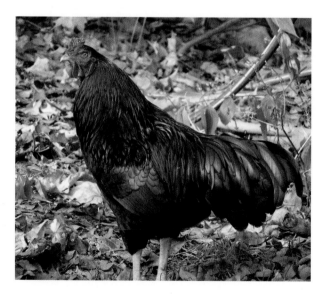

Figure 14.11 Cornish. *Source*: Courtesy of Wendy MacDonald.

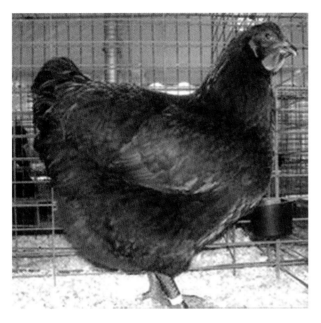

Figure 14.12 Jersey Giant.

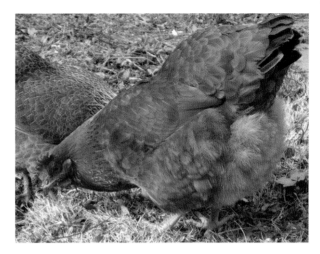

Figure 14.14 New Hampshire Red.

an Italian breed that is primarily an egg-laying breed that produces white-shelled eggs. It is similar in appearance to the Leghorn, which also originated in Italy and is known for its high egg-laying capacity. It is one of the most popular egg-producing chicken breeds in the United States and has 16 different varieties by color and comb type. The Andalusian was developed in the Spanish province of Andalusia and is a blue-colored and a medium-sized bird that produces white-shelled eggs. The Brahma was developed in China and bred specifically as a meat breed; it produces brown-shelled eggs and has feathered legs. The Buckeye originated in Ohio and is a dual-purpose breed and is dark brown in color. The Catalana was developed in Spain and is a large, buff-colored, dual-purpose bird that produces white- to lightly tinted brown-shelled eggs. The Cochin is a popular breed of Chinese origin known for its soft plumage that creates a lot of volume over the body and produces an illusion of great size (Figure 14.10). Cochins have feathers on their legs and produce brown-shelled eggs. Originally a meat breed, they are now bred primarily for exhibition. The Cornish was developed in England as a primary meat-producing bird and is used heavily in cross-breeding market poultry (Figure 14.11). It is small in size and lays brown-shelled eggs. The Delaware originated in the United States by crossing barred Plymouth Rocks and New Hampshire Reds. It is a dual-purpose breed that grows quickly and is used in broiler production and produces large brown

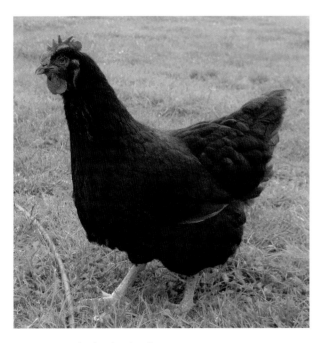

Figure 14.13 Rhode Island Red.

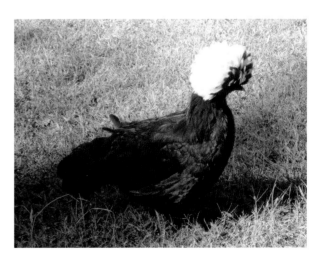

Figure 14.15 Polish.

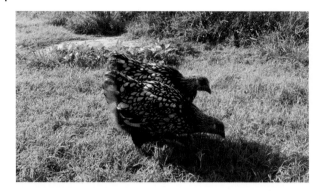

Figure 14.16 Wyandotte.

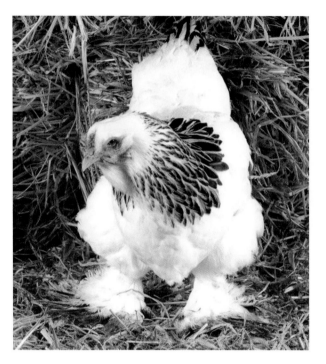

Figure 14.17 Bantam.

eggs. The Holland chicken is a heavy, dual-purpose breed that produces white-shelled eggs and was developed from a variety of other popular chicken breeds.

The Jersey Giant is the largest of the chicken breeds that was developed in the United States with an emphasis on creating a large meat-producing bird with a dual purpose in producing brown-shelled eggs (Figure 14.12). The Langshan breed was developed in China as a dual-purpose bird that has feathered legs and produces dark brown-shelled eggs. The Rhode Island Red was developed in the United States by crossing several Asiatic breeds and is dark red in color with black markings. It is a dual-purpose breed that produces brown-shelled eggs (Figure 14.13). The New Hampshire Red was developed from Rhode Island stock and is lighter red in color but otherwise similar to the Rhode Island Red (Figure 14.14). It is more common in broiler production systems.

The Plymouth Rock breed was one of the first breeds to be admitted into the APA *Standard of Perfection* and is a dual-purpose breed that produces brown-shelled eggs and used mainly in cross-breeding programs to develop commercial broilers. The Polish was developed in Eastern Europe primarily as an ornamental type (Figure 14.15). The unique feature is the head, which has

Figure 14.18 Bronze.

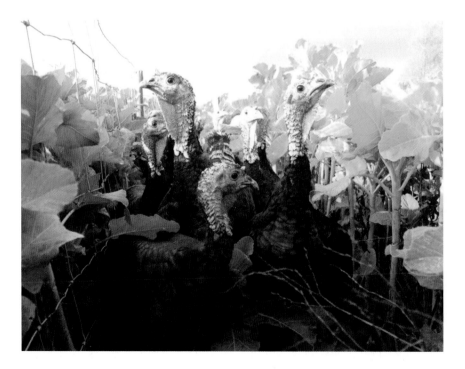

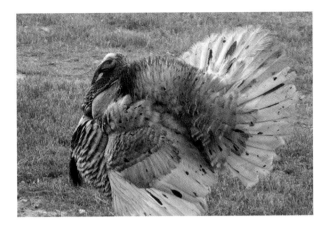

Figure 14.19 Slate.

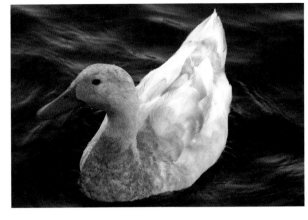

Figure 14.21 Buff.

a crested appearance and develops feathers around the face and head that may form a beard, cap, or ear muff appearance. There are 11 varieties based on beard and color. These birds produce white-shelled eggs. The Redcap originated in England and is characterized by a large rosecomb and is known for its high production of white-shelled eggs. The Spanish breed is one of the oldest Mediterranean breeds. These chickens are black in body color with a unique white coloration of the face. The Sultan is an ancient ornamental breed developed in Turkey and has unique feathering on the face, legs, and toes. It is white in color and produces white-shelled eggs. The Sussex was developed in England as a dual-purpose breed

with an emphasis on meat production. They produce brown-shelled eggs. The Wyandotte originated in New York with a silver to white color and is a dual-purpose breed that produces brown-shelled eggs (Figure 14.16). Bantam chickens are one fourth to one fifth the size of standard chicken breeds (Figure 14.17). They have a disproportionately large head in relation to their body, wings, and tails. Weight is the only difference in their varieties and the common Bantams include Silkie, Dutch, Japanese, Belgian, Rosecomb, and Booted.

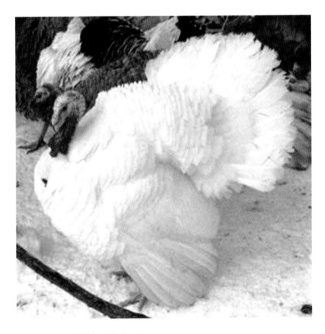

Figure 14.20 White Holland.

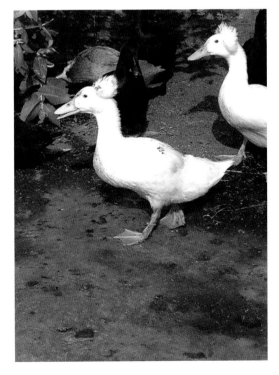

Figure 14.22 Crested.

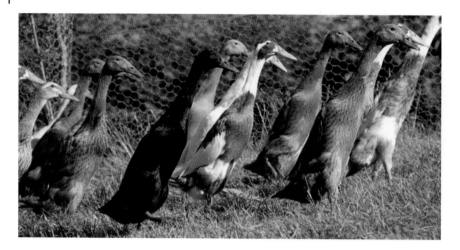

Figure 14.23 Indian Runner.

14.4.2 Turkey Breeds

The Black turkey is solid black in color; males weigh over 30 pounds and females around 18 pounds. The Bronze turkey is commonly seen as a wild domesticated turkey that is very similar to the coppery bronze shades of a wild turkey (Figure 14.18). The male weighs over 35 pounds and the female around 20 pounds. The Royal Palm turkey has distinctive white feathers tipped in black. The male weighs over 20 pounds and the female around 12 pounds. The Slate turkey is slate blue in color and males weigh over 30 pounds and females around 18 pounds (Figure 14.19). The White Holland turkey is the most commonly raised commercial turkey breed and may also be known as a large white or broad white (Figure 14.20). Males weigh over 35 pounds and females around 20 pounds.

14.4.3 Duck Breeds

The Aylesbury duck is a large, heavyweight, white bird weighing over 10 pounds that was developed in England and has a flesh-colored bill and white skin. It is popular in England as a meat production duck. The Buff is a medium-weight breed of around 8 pounds and has a uniform buff color (Figure 14.21). The Campbell is a lightweight breed of around 4 pounds with a dark green bill and brown- to tan-colored feathers. The Crested is a medium-sized breed that has a unique pattern of feathers on the top of the head (Figure 14.22). The Indian Runner was developed in India and is characterized by a long, pencil-thin neck and narrow and cylindrical body that moves upright in posture (Figure 14.23). The Magpie is a lightweight breed of around 5 pounds that is primarily white with blue or black feathers on the top of the head, on the back, and on the tail. The Pekin is a popular large Chinese duck breed of over 10 pounds in weight that is white with a bright orange beak. They are raised

primarily for meat in the United States. The Muscovy is a heavyweight breed from South America that is distinctive in having fleshy knobbed skin around the eyes and face (Figure 14.24). The Swedish duck is a medium-sized blue-feathered breed that has a blue bill and is favorable in meat production.

14.4.4 Goose Breeds

The African goose is a large, heavyweight goose that has a large knob on the base of the beak where it joins the head. The color of the knob varies by the type of goose. The Canada goose is a common wild lightweight goose breed that is gray and black in body color with black legs and bill and weighs around 12 pounds (Figure 14.25). The Embden is a heavyweight breed that is solid white with a broad orange bill. The Egyptian goose is a lightweight breed that is reddish brown, gray, and black in color (Figure 14.26). The Pilgrim is a medium-sized goose breed with colors relating to gender differences (Figure 14.27). The male is creamy white and the female is olive gray. The Toulouse is a large breed that is gray or buff in color with a flat bill and a dewlap extending from the bottom of the jaw to the neck. The White Chinese or Chinese goose is a lightweight breed of around 10 pounds that is bred specifically as an ornament (Figure 14.28). They have a short body, long neck, and distinctive knob on the base of the bill where it joins the head. They are white or brown in color.

14.4.5 Ratite Species

The common ratites that are raised for production include the ostrich, which is the most commonly recognized flightless bird (Figure 14.29). It can grow up to 6 feet tall and over 400 pounds in weight and was developed in

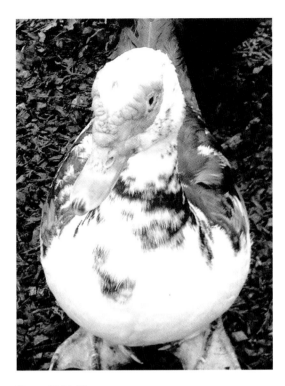

Figure 14.24 Muscovy.

Africa. It was originally domesticated for feather production in the 1800s but now is a source of meat, eggs, feathers, oils, and other by-products. The color of ostrich is gender specific, with males being black in body color and females light gray. Ostriches have a long, thin neck and long, powerful legs and feet. They are the largest bird in the world. The emu is another large, flightless bird native to Australia that is often raised for meat and eggs (Figure 14.30). They are the second largest bird in the world and are grayish brown in body color with black-tipped feathers. They are around 5 feet tall and 120 pounds in weight and males tend to be smaller than females. The rhea is native to South America and stands around 4–4.5

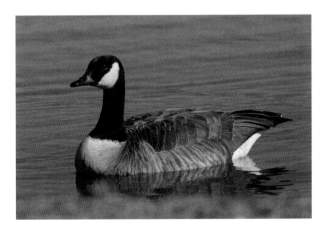

Figure 14.25 Canada goose.

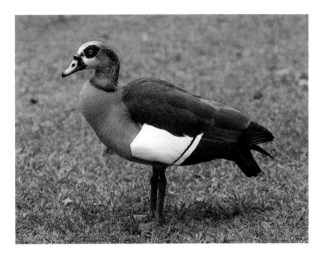

Figure 14.26 Egyptian goose.

feet tall and weighs about 80 pounds (Figure 14.31). The body color is light gray brown to white and the rhea has no tail feathers.

> ***Points to remember.*** Ratites are large, flightless birds.

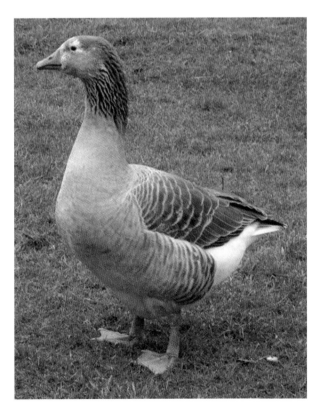

Figure 14.27 Pilgrim.

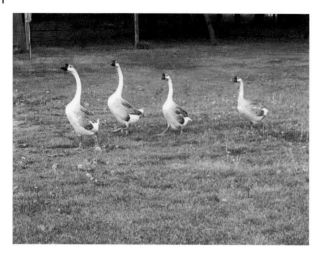

Figure 14.28 White Chinese.

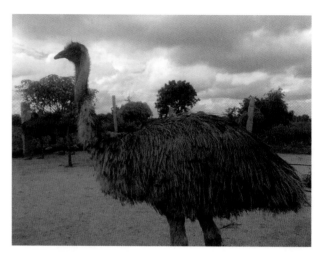

Figure 14.30 Emu.

14.4.6 Other Poultry Species

Other common poultry production breeds include the guinea fowl, which is a small, game-type bird raised for eggs and as a hobby (Figure 14.32). It has a distinctive appearance in which it looks rather prehistoric with an oversized body and short, thin head and neck. The color varies from shades of dark gray to black with white speckles. The peafowl is often called the peacock, which is actually the male term for the species (Figure 14.33). It is strictly an ornamental bird that is blue to green in color and the male has a distinctive long tail plumage with markings like an "eye" when the train is open and spread. The pigeon is a small bird raised for hobby

Figure 14.29 Ostrich.

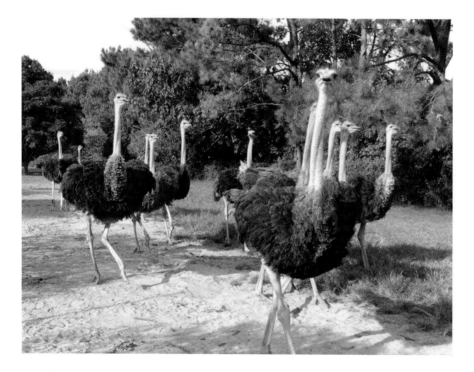

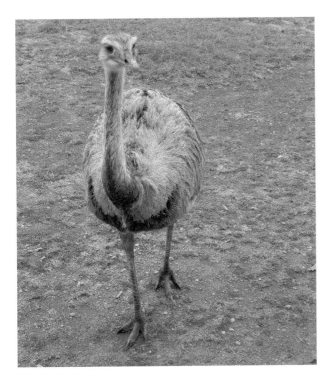

Figure 14.31 Rhea.

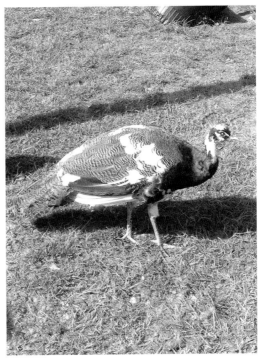

Figure 14.33 Peafowl.

14.5 Summary

purposes such as showing or racing (Figure 14.34). It has a small, round body that is gray in color and has a small head. Several color varieties have been developed. The quail is another type of game bird that has been raised for meat and eggs. The colors are gender specific, with the male having a gray body with brown markings on the chest and black markings on the head and the female having a brown camouflage color.

Chickens, ducks, turkeys, geese, ratites, and some game birds are considered as poultry and may be raised for their meat, eggs, feathers, hides, and other by-products depending on species. The poultry industry is widespread, with the American Poultry Association recognizing over 400 breeds and varieties of birds. Knowledge of the differences in poultry species aids in identifying the types of commonly raised production animals.

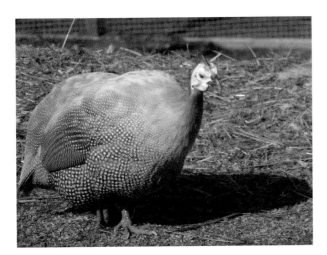

Figure 14.32 Guinea fowl.

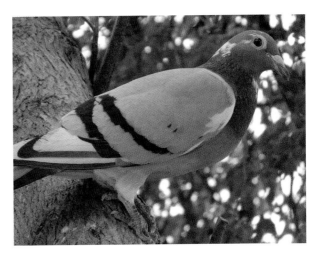

Figure 14.34 Pigeon.

Sources

American Poultry Association (APA) (2016).

American Poultry Association (2010) *The American Standard of Perfection*, American Poultry Association, Burgettstown, PA.

USDA (2012) *2012 National Agricultural Statistics Service Survey*, United States Department of Agriculture, Washington, DC.

Further Reading

Damerow, G. (2012) *The Chicken Encyclopedia*, Storey Publishing, North Adams, MA.

Ekarius, C. (2016) *Storey's Illustrated Guide to Poultry Breeds*, Storey Publishing, North Adams, MA.

Hams, F. (2015) *The Concise Encyclopedia of Poultry Breeds*, Southwater, London.

15

Alternative Production Animal Breed Identification

15.1 Introduction

Although several types of common livestock dominate the production animal industry, a growing number of alternative animal species operations are producing other animals for consumption and by-products. Knowledge and marketing of these animals are very important to the producer as a focal point on the differences in nutrients and meat sources. Alternative production systems include aquaculture, namely fish and shellfish farming. Other common mammals have also become increasingly popular as alternative production animals.

15.2 Alternative Animal Production Systems

15.2.1 Aquaculture

Aquaculture is the practice of raising fish, shellfish, and other water-related sea life for human consumption (Figure 15.1). A wide variety of aquatic and semi-aquatic species are raised for production, but food fish is the largest component of the aquaculture industry. Species may be raised as food, bait, or stock.

15.2.2 Bison

Bison have been a growing popular source of nutritious meat (Figure 15.2). Sometimes called buffalo, these are tamed wild animals that can be extremely territorial and aggressive, especially in the breeding season. Bison have not been bred in captivity long enough to be considered a domesticated animal. The management of bison is similar to that of cattle. Bison produce red meat that is lower in fat, calories, and cholesterol than beef.

15.2.3 Deer

Cervidae is the broad term used to describe many types of deer that are raised for meat production (Figure 15.3). Regulations controlling the species and use of farmed deer vary between local and state laws. Deer may be raised as trophy deer for hunting and others for meat production, called venison. Varieties of deer raised within the United States can be divided into native and non-native species.

15.2.4 Camelids

Camelids are a type of pack animal native to South America. They were domesticated in Peru around 4000 years ago and are raised for multiple purposes, including food, fiber, guard animals, show animals, pets, and pack animals. Camelids include alpacas and llamas that were brought to the United States in the 1800s as unique animals added to zoos (Figure 15.4). They began to find a place in agriculture in the 1970s.

15.3 Common Alternative Production Animal Species

15.3.1 Aquaculture Species

Aquaculture species include bass, such as the largemouth bass raised primarily for sport fish that are released into recreational water and fishing areas. Catfish species represent the largest farming production system in the United States (Figure 15.5). Catfish are known for their white, firm meat with a mild taste and few bones. There

Veterinary Guide to Animal Breeds, First Edition. Beth Vanhorn.
© 2018 John Wiley & Sons, Inc. Published 2018 by John Wiley & Sons, Inc.
Companion website: www.wiley.com/go/vanhorn/breeds

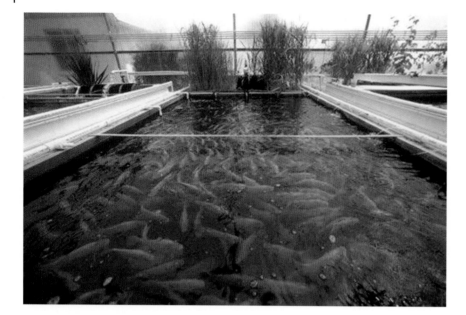

Figure 15.1 Aquaculture production system.

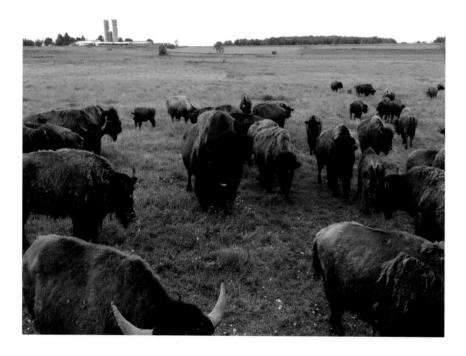

Figure 15.2 Bison farm.

Figure 15.3 Deer farm.

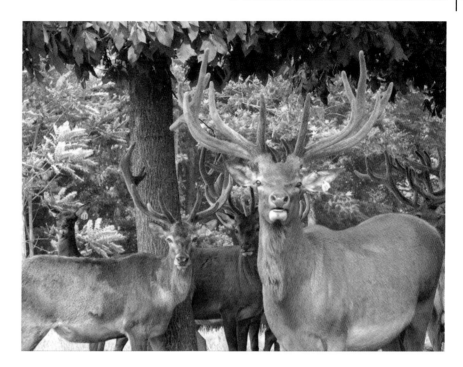

Figure 15.4 Alpaca farm.

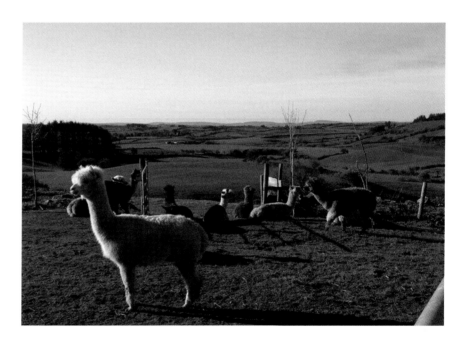

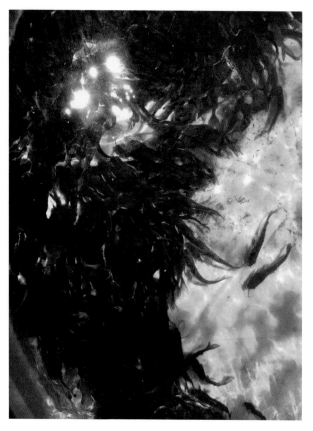

Figure 15.5 Catfish farming.

is a market for both food fish production and stocking as sport fish. Salmon are large fish with reddish flesh that are farmed most commonly in Washington and Maine (Figure 15.6). Several varieties of salmon are raised both as food fish and as fish stock. Tilapia is a white fish raised for the commercial fish market. Trout is a game fish species that has had the longest production time in the aquaculture setting (Figure 15.7). Trout are medium-sized fish that are raised as food fish and for restocking fishing sites.

15.3.2 Bison Production

Bison are characterized by dark brown to black body colors, with a pronounced hump over the shoulder area and a body that tapers toward the hindquarters. Mature bulls weigh over 2000 pounds and cows around 1000 pounds. There has been cross-breeding with cattle and bison to develop the beefalo (Figure 15.8).

15.3.3 Deer Production

Deer production systems may include native and non-native species. Non-native species are those not naturally found within the United States, and include Axis deer, raised primarily for trophy hunting and venison production. They are native to India and have a bright reddish

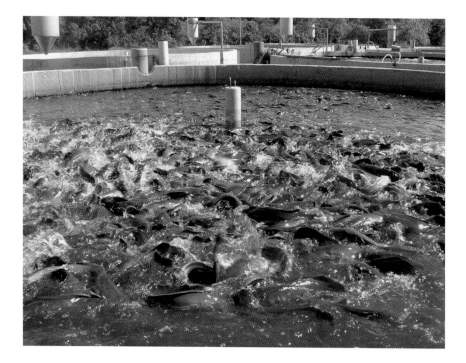

Figure 15.6 Salmon farming.

Figure 15.7 Trout farming.

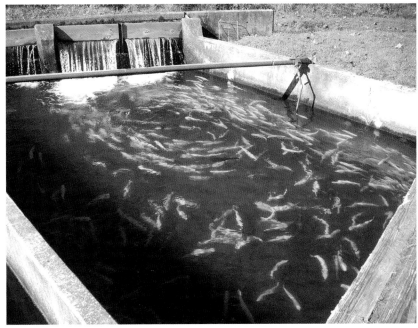

Figure 15.8 Beefalo.

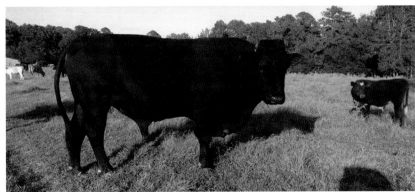

Figure 15.9 Fallow deer.

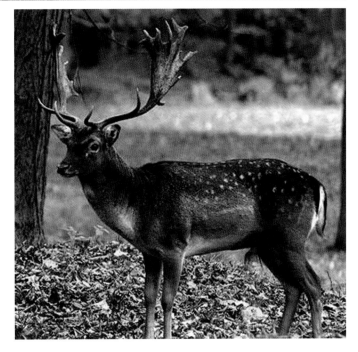

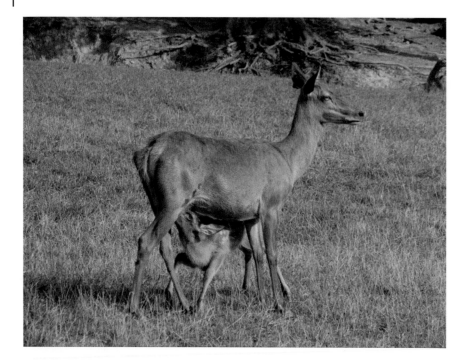

Figure 15.10 Red deer.

coat color marked with row of white spots that are visible for the deer's entire adult life. Fallow deer are primarily raised for venison (Figure 15.9). They are light cream to chestnut in color with some white spots visible in the summer. Red deer are a relatively large species raised for venison and velvet (Figure 15.10). They are native to Europe and Asia, are red in color and may weigh over 500 pounds. They are known for having longer tails than many deer species. Sika deer are also relatively large and are raised primarily for venison (Figure 15.11). They are native to Eastern Asia and are also known as Japanese deer. They can weigh around 200 pounds and have a fawn to red body color with large white spots over the hair coat.

Native species include White-Tailed deer that are farmed primarily as trophy animals (Figure 15.12). They are commonly called the Whitetail and are a medium-sized deer found in North America with a reddish brown to gray brown coat color depending on the season. They have a characteristic white underside to the tail that when raised flashes white. Elk are the largest deer species native to North America (Figure 15.13). They are raised for meat, trophy, and velvet. They are light brown in body color with a darker neck. Elk can weigh over 500 pounds.

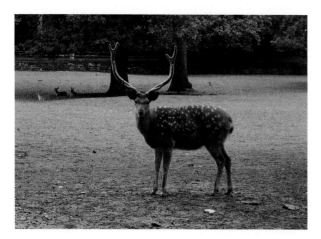

Figure 15.11 Sika deer.

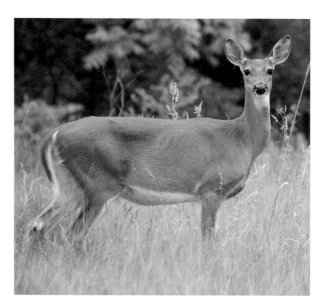

Figure 15.12 White-Tailed deer.

Figure 15.13 Elk.

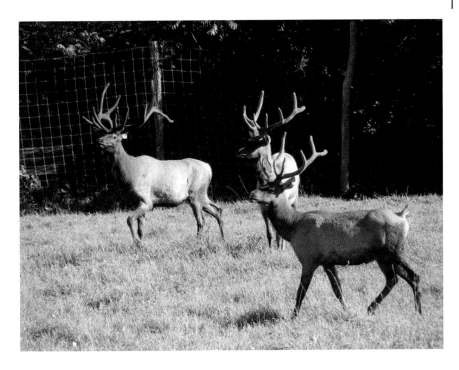

15.3.4 Pack Animal Production

The common domesticated camelids include the alpaca, which is a small ruminant animal from South America that has short, pointed ears and may weigh up to 175 pounds (Figure 15.14). An alpaca can produce up to 4 pounds of hair per year. They are found in a range of colors and color combinations and are raised primarily for their fleece and showing and as pets. The Huacaya alpaca breed has crimped fleece and is the most common breed found in the United States. The Suri alpaca breed has long and wavy fleece that can grow to the ground. The llama is a larger ruminant animal from South America with banana-shaped ears and found in a variety of colors and combinations (Figure 15.15). Adults can weigh up to 450 pounds. They are used as pack animals, for showing, and for fleece that is sheared to make cloth. Llama fleece is coarser than that of alpacas. Llamas are

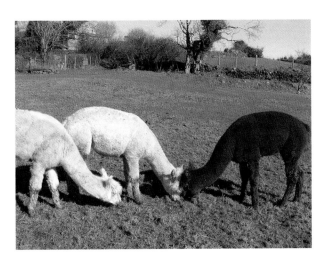

Figure 15.14 Alpaca.

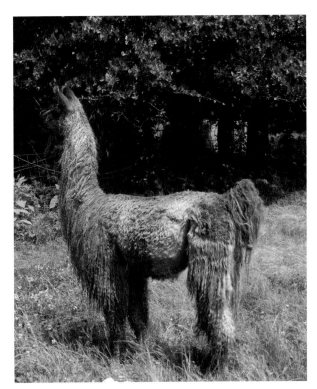

Figure 15.15 Llama.

very protective and can serve as guard animals to sheep and other livestock.

15.4 Summary

Although cattle, sheep, and goats may be traditional species of production animals, a variety of other species have developed a role in the industry. Markets exist for non-traditional types of animals that serve as sources of food, fiber, and other products. The primary market is for consumers who are interested in alternative low-fat meat. Knowledge of certain animal species that are utilized in this alternative industry will aid in identifying specific species and breeds.

Sources

Alpaca Llama Show Association (2016).
National Bison Association (2016).
United States Department of Agriculture (2016).
USDA (2012) *2012 National Agricultural Statistics Service Survey*, United States Department of Agriculture, Washington, DC.

Further Reading

Gegner, L. and Sharp, H. (2012) *Llamas and Alpacas on the Farm*, National Sustainable Agriculture Information Service, National Center for Appropriate Technology, Butte, MT.
Lantz, D.E. (2012) *Raising Deer and Other Large Game Animals in the United States*, Nabu Press, Charleston, SC (originally published 1910).

Appendix

Table A1 United States census of domestic animals.

Dogs	Cats	Rabbits	Ferrets	Hamsters	Pigs
69,926,000	74,059,000	3,210,000	748,000	1,146,000	62,485,647
Lizards	**Horses**	**Dairy cows**	**Beef cows**	**Poultry**	**Sheep**
1,119,000	1,780,000	9,300,000	619,172	12,591,000	6,200,000
Birds	**Guinea pigs**	**Gerbils**	**Turtles**	**Snakes**	**Goats**
3,671,000	1,362,000	468,000	2,297,000	1,150,000	750,000

Sources:

AVMA (2012) *U.S. Pet Ownership & Demographics Sourcebook*, American Veterinary Medical Association, Schaumburg, IL.

USDA (2012) *2012 National Agricultural Statistics Service Survey*, United States Department of Agriculture, Washington, DC.

Photographs of Animal Breeds

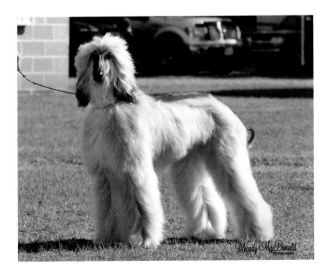

Figure A1 Afghan Hound. *Source*: Courtesy of Wendy MacDonald.

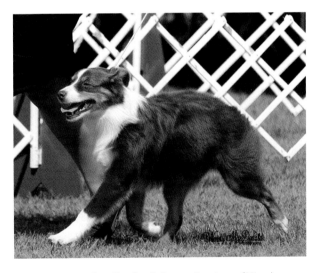

Figure A2 Australian Shepherd. *Source*: Courtesy of Wendy MacDonald.

Veterinary Guide to Animal Breeds, First Edition. Beth Vanhorn.
© 2018 John Wiley & Sons, Inc. Published 2018 by John Wiley & Sons, Inc.
Companion website: www.wiley.com/go/vanhorn/breeds

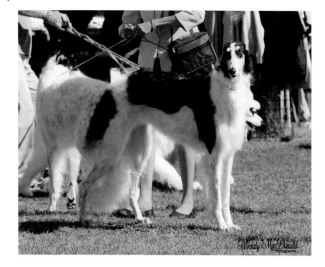

Figure A3 Borzoi. *Source*: Courtesy of Wendy MacDonald.

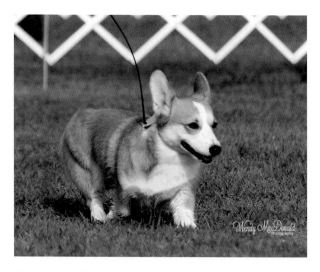

Figure A6 Pembroke Welsh Corgi. *Source*: Courtesy of Wendy MacDonald.

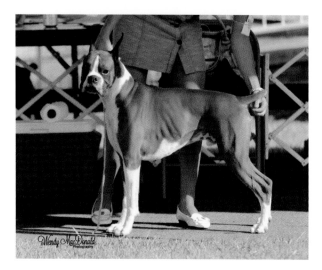

Figure A4 Boxer. *Source*: Courtesy of Wendy MacDonald.

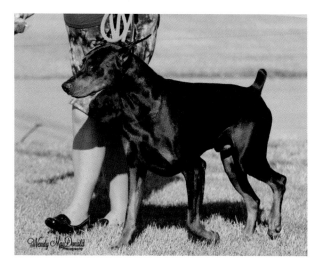

Figure A7 Doberman Pinscher. *Source*: Courtesy of Wendy MacDonald.

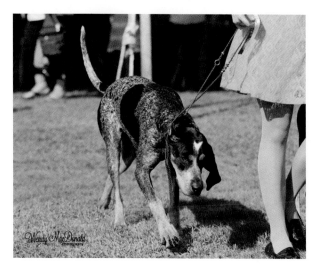

Figure A5 Bluetick Coonhound. *Source*: Courtesy of Wendy MacDonald.

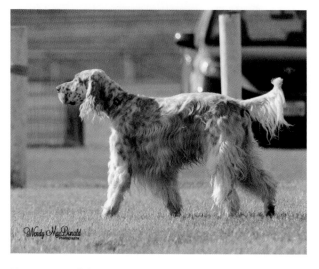

Figure A8 English Setter. *Source*: Courtesy of Wendy MacDonald.

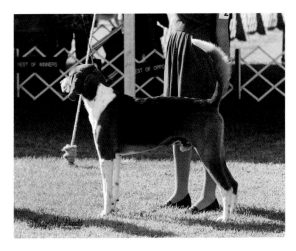

Figure A9 American Foxhound. *Source*: Courtesy of Wendy MacDonald.

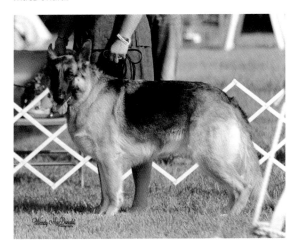

Figure A10 German Shepherd Dog. *Source*: Courtesy of Wendy MacDonald.

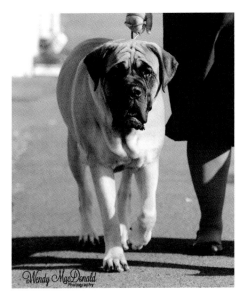

Figure A11 Mastiff. *Source*: Courtesy of Wendy MacDonald.

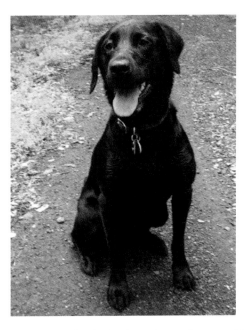

Figure A12 Labrador Retriever. *Source*: Courtesy of Sarah Moyer.

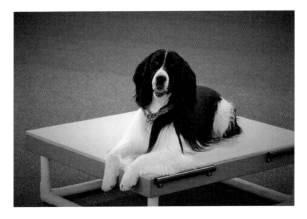

Figure A13 English Springer Spaniel. *Source*: Courtesy of Shari Krause.

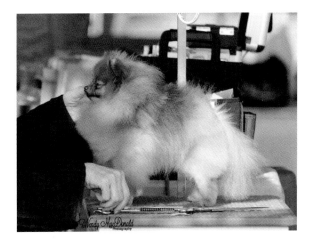

Figure A14 Pomeranian. *Source*: Courtesy of Wendy MacDonald.

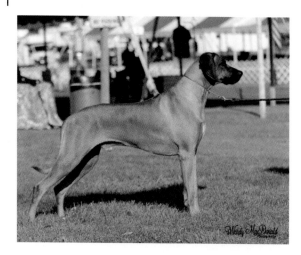

Figure A15 Rhodesian Ridgeback. *Source*: Courtesy of Wendy MacDonald.

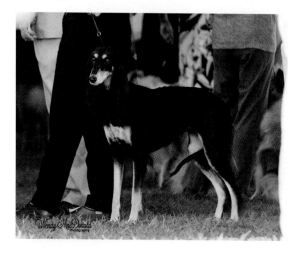

Figure A16 Saluki. *Source*: Courtesy of Wendy MacDonald.

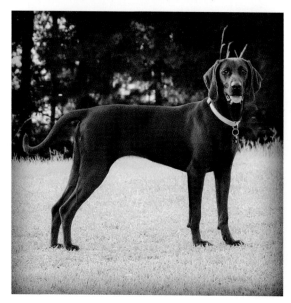

Figure A17 Redbone Coonhound.

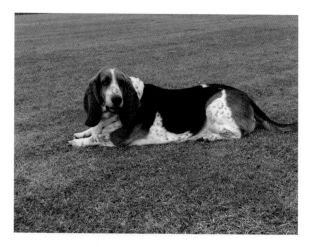

Figure A18 Basset Hound.

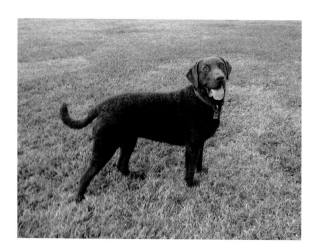

Figure A19 Chesapeake Bay Retriever.

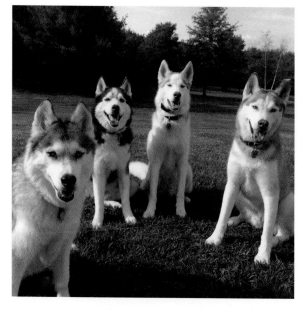

Figure A20 Siberian Husky. *Source*: Courtesy of Sonya Rothermel.

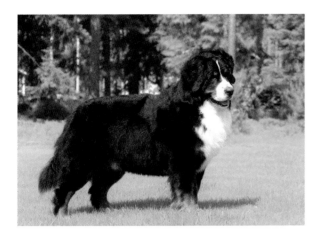

Figure A21 Bernese Mountain Dog.

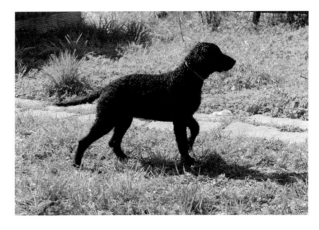

Figure A24 Curly Coated Retriever.

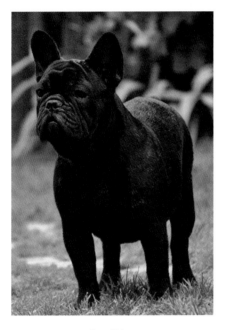

Figure A22 French Bulldog.

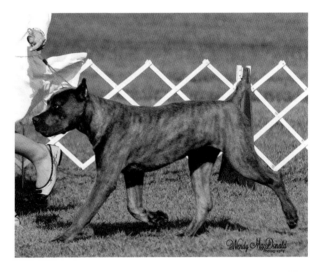

Figure A25 Cane Corso. *Source*: Courtesy of Wendy MacDonald.

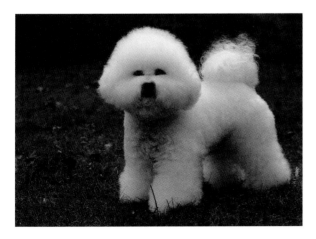

Figure A23 Bichon Frise.

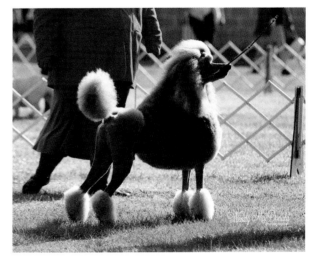

Figure A26 Standard Poodle. *Source*: Courtesy of Wendy MacDonald.

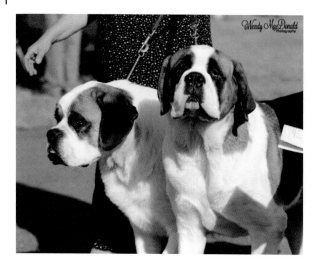

Figure A27 Saint Bernard.

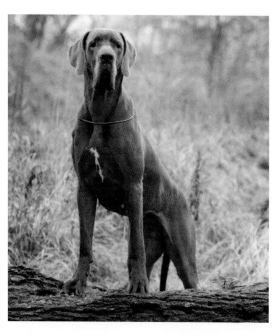

Figure A28 Great Dane.

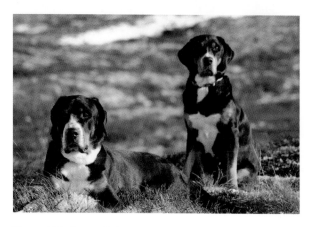

Figure A29 Greater Swiss Mountain Dog.

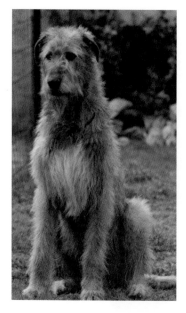

Figure A30 Irish Wolfhound.

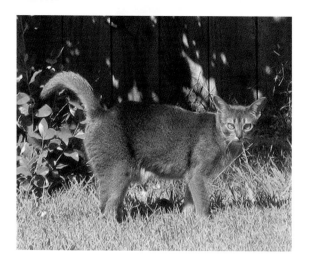

Figure A31 Abyssinian.

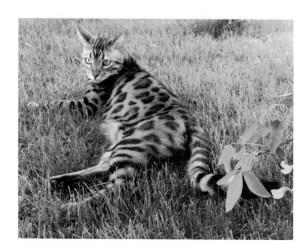

Figure A32 Bengal.

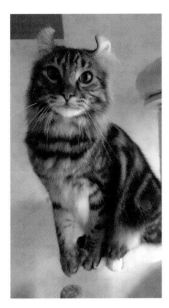

Figure A33 American Curl.

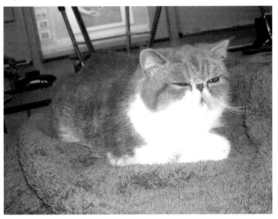

Figure A34 Exotic.

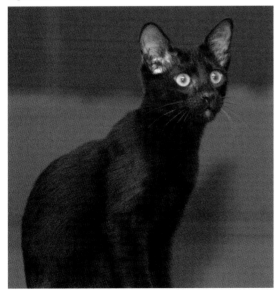

Figure A35 Havana Brown.

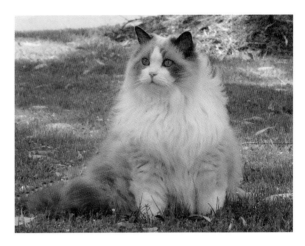

Figure A36 Himalayan.

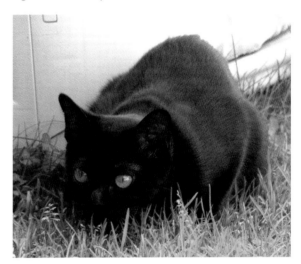

Figure A37 Bombay.

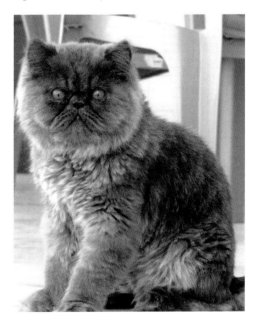

Figure A38 Persian.

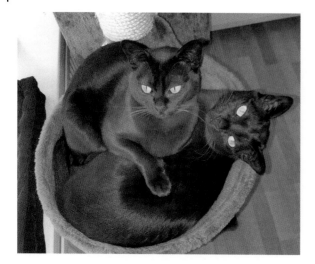

Figure A39 Burmese.

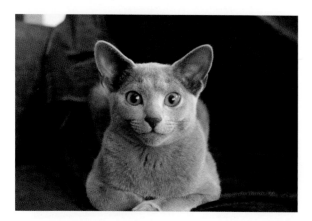

Figure A40 Russian Blue.

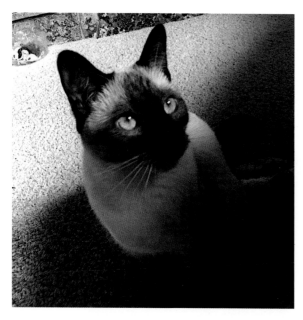

Figure A41 Siamese.

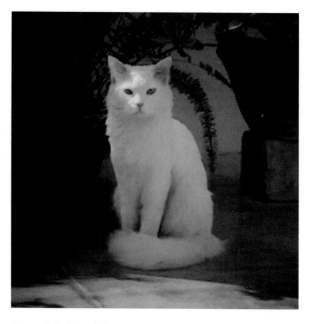

Figure A42 Turkish Angora.

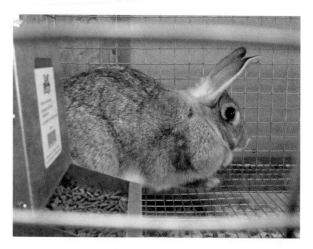

Figure A43 American Chinchilla.

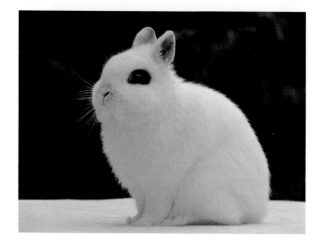

Figure A44 Dwarf Hotot.

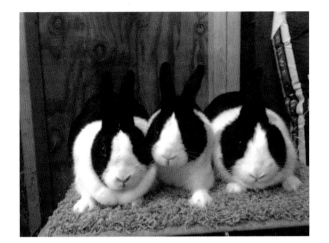

Figure A45 Dutch.

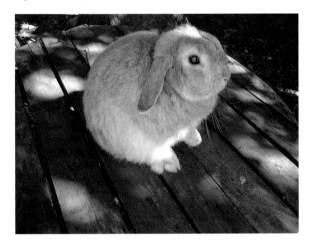

Figure A46 Holland Lop.

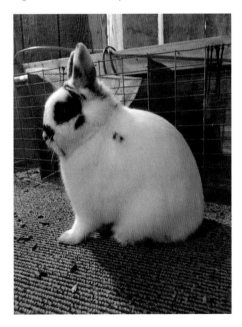

Figure A47 Netherland Dwarf.

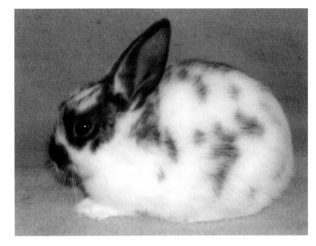

Figure A48 Polish.

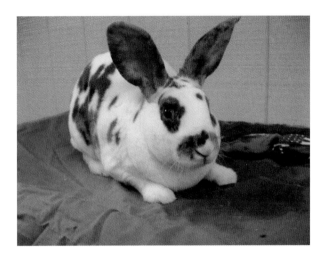

Figure A49 Rex.

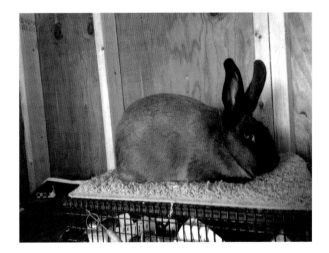

Figure A50 American Sable.

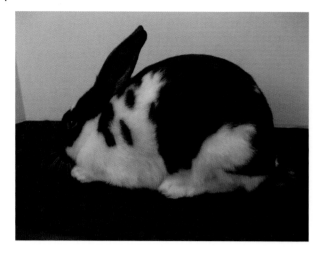

Figure A51 Satin.

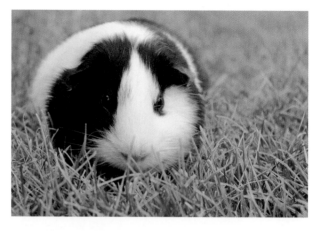

Figure A54 American.

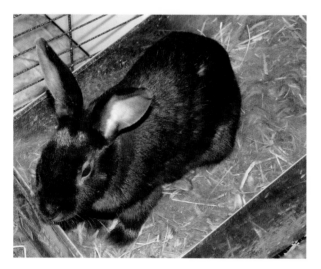

Figure A52 Tan.

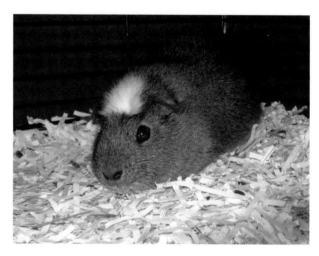

Figure A55 White Crested.

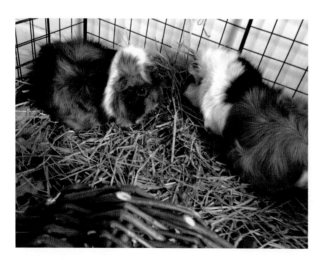

Figure A53 Abyssinian.

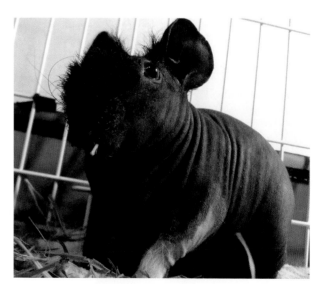

Figure A56 Skinny.

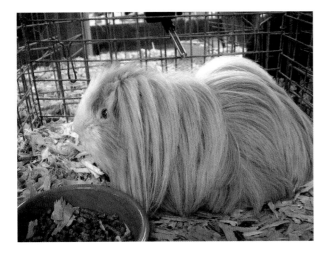

Figure A57 Peruvian.

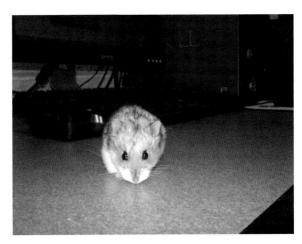

Figure A60 Russian Dwarf Hamster.

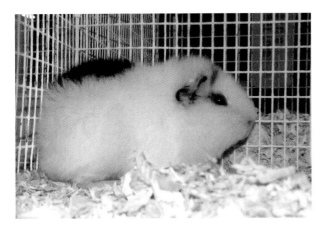

Figure A58 Teddy.

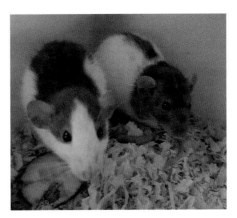

Figure A61 Dumbo Rat.

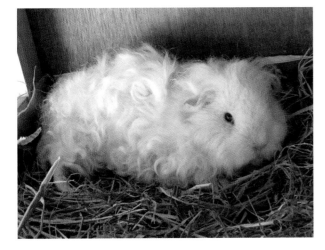

Figure A59 Texel.

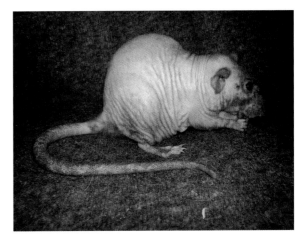

Figure A62 Hairless Rat.

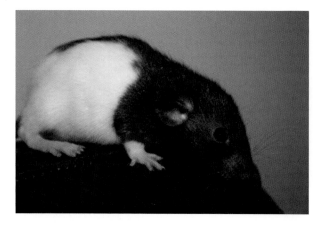

Figure A63 Hooded Rat.

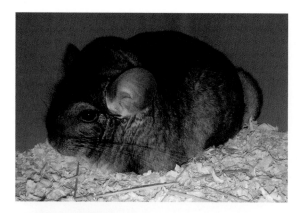

Figure A66 Chinchilla.

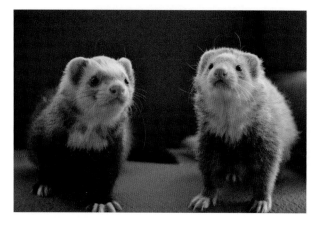

Figure A64 Ferret.

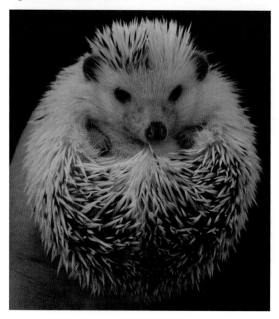

Figure A67 Hedgehog.

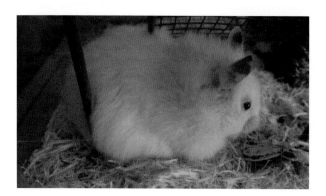

Figure A65 Teddy Bear Hamster.

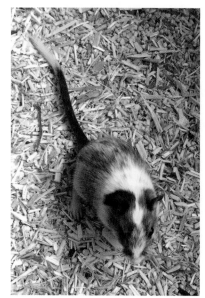

Figure A68 Gerbil.

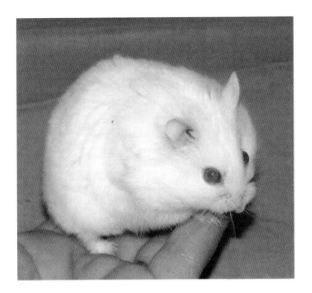

Figure A69 Winter White Hamster.

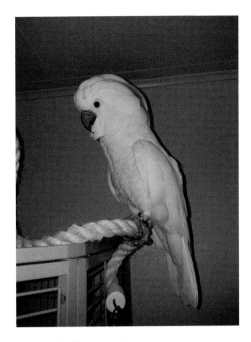

Figure A72 Moluccan Cockatoo.

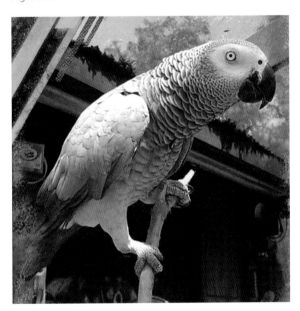

Figure A70 African Grey Parrot.

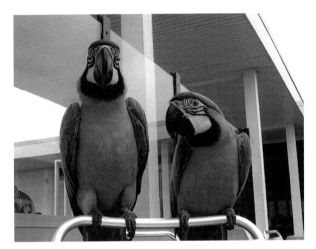

Figure A73 Blue and Gold Macaw.

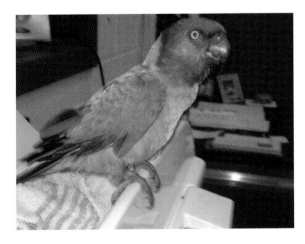

Figure A71 Senegal Parrot.

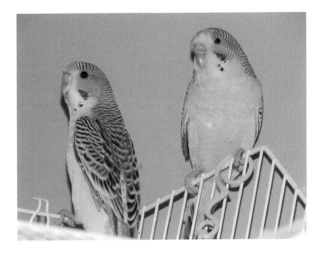

Figure A74 Budgerigar/Parakeet.

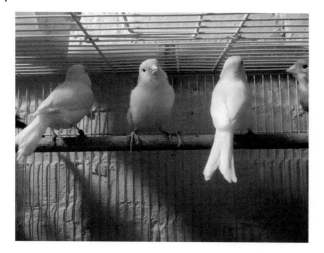

Figure A75 Canary.

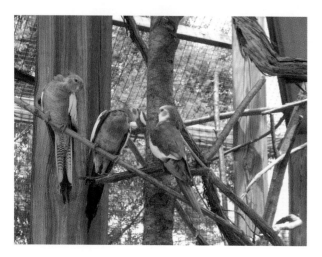

Figure A76 Cockatiel.

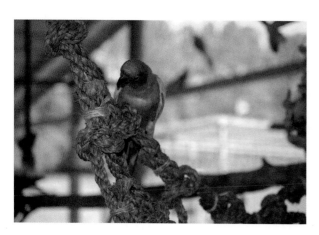

Figure A77 Sun Conure.

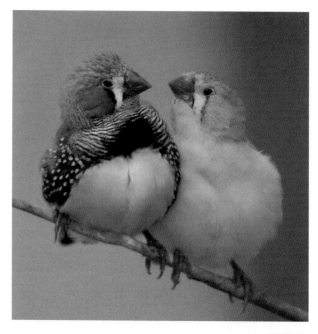

Figure A78 Zebra Finch.

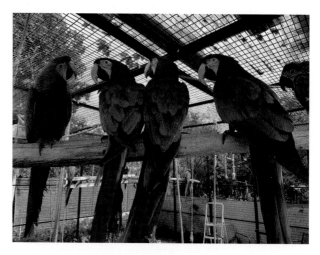

Figure A79 Green Winged Macaw.

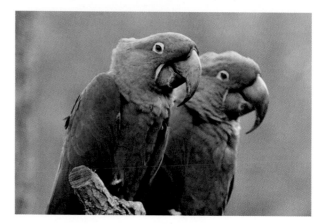

Figure A80 Hyacinth Macaw.

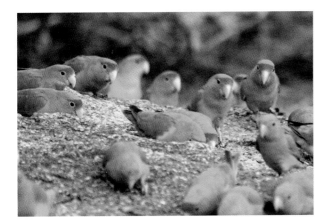

Figure A81 Peach Faced Lovebird.

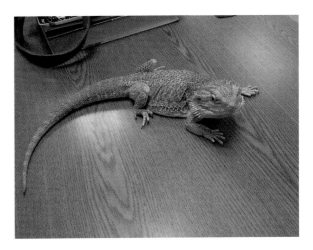

Figure A84 Bearded Dragon.

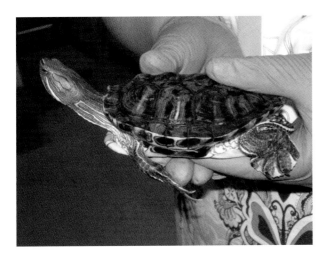

Figure A82 Red Ear Slider.

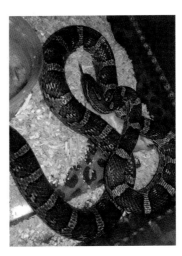

Figure A85 Corn Snake.

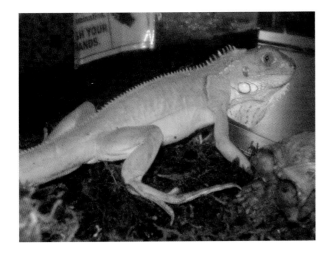

Figure A83 Green Iguana.

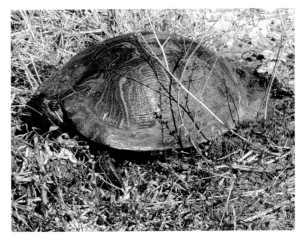

Figure A86 Map Turtle.

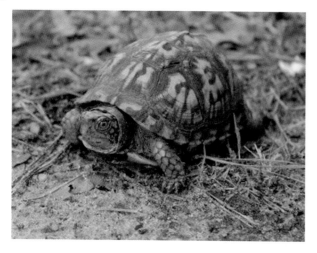

Figure A87 Box Turtle.

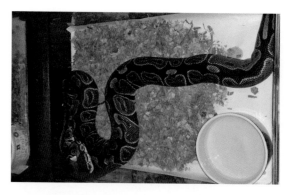

Figure A90 Ball Python.

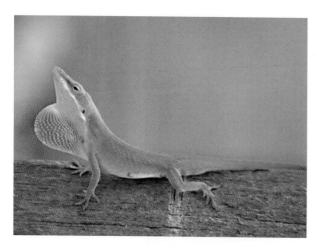

Figure A88 Green Anole.

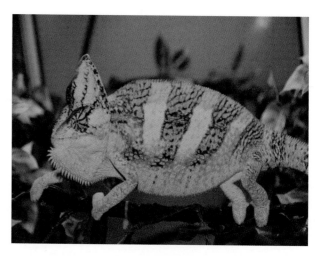

Figure A91 Veiled Chameleon.

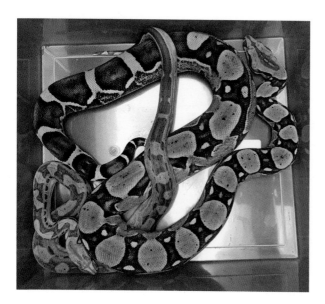

Figure A89 Boa Constrictor.

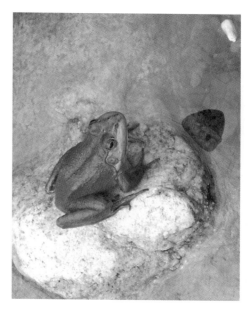

Figure A92 American Bullfrog.

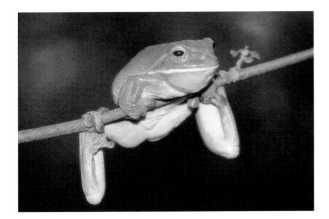

Figure A93 Green Treefrog.

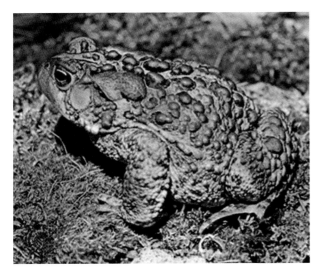

Figure A94 American Toad.

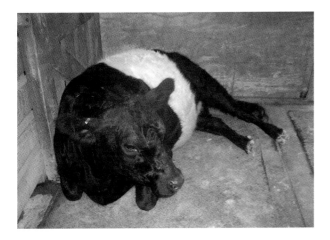

Figure A95 Galloway.

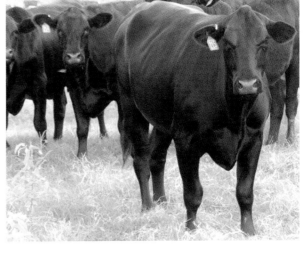

Figure A96 Angus.

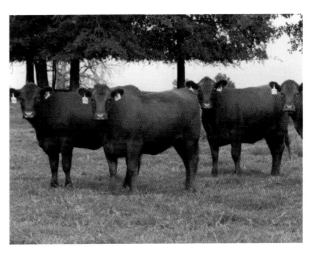

Figure A97 Red Angus.

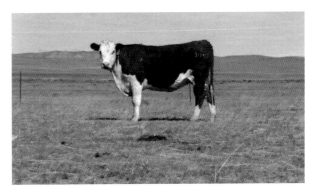

Figure A98 Hereford.

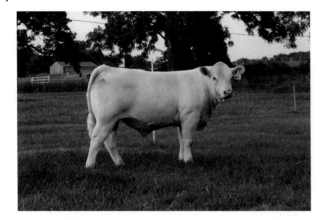

Figure A99 Charolais.

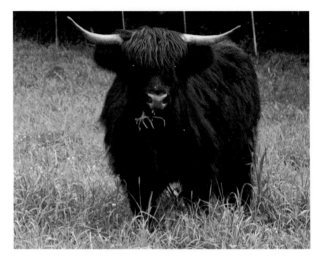

Figure A102 Highland.

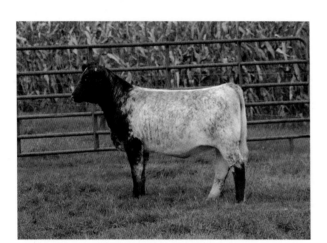

Figure A100 Shorthorn.

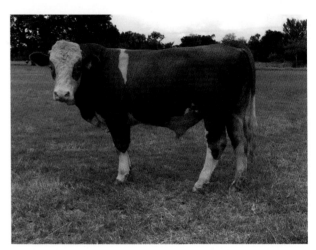

Figure A103 Simmental.

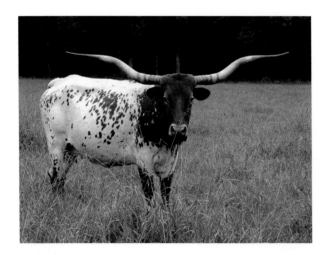

Figure A101 Texas Longhorn.

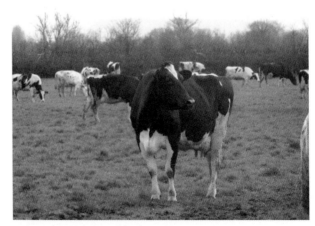

Figure A104 Holstein.

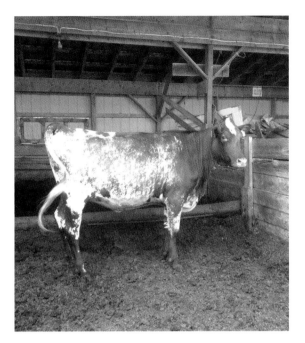

Figure A105   Milking Shorthorn.

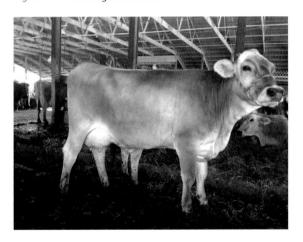

Figure A106   Brown Swiss.

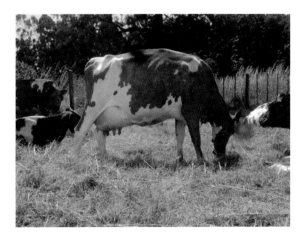

Figure A107   Guernsey.

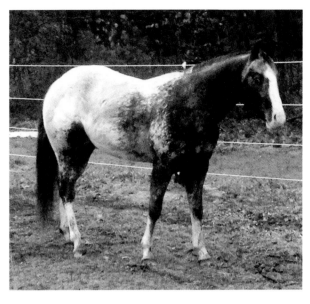

Figure A108   Appaloosa.

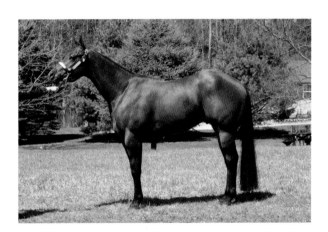

Figure A109   American Quarter Horse.

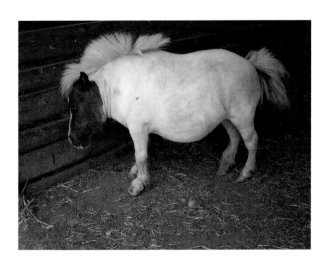

Figure A110   American Miniature Horse.

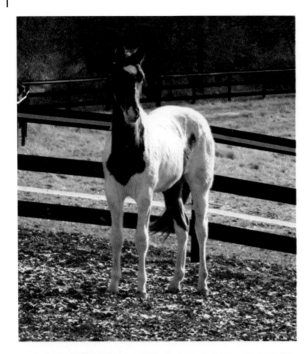

Figure A111 Paint. *Source*: Courtesy of Amanda Reed.

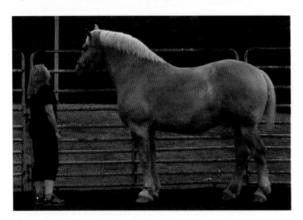

Figure A112 Belgian. *Source*: Courtesy of Shari Krause.

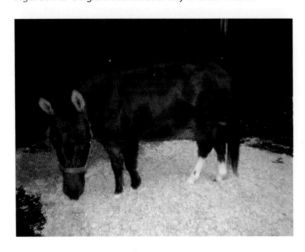

Figure A113 Miniature Mule.

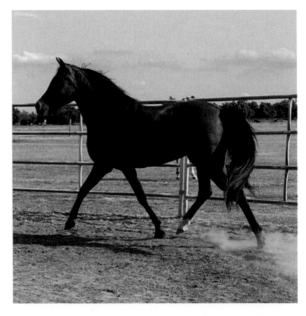

Figure A114 Arabian.

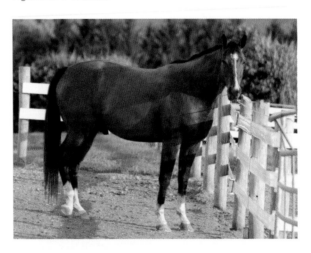

Figure A115 Thoroughbred.

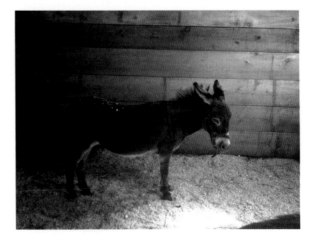

Figure A116 Donkey.

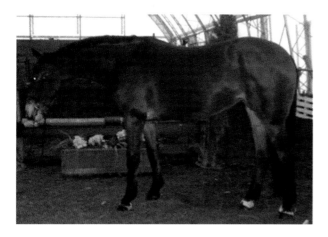

Figure A117   Hanoverian. *Source*: Courtesy of Jessica Berman.

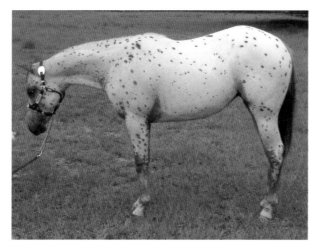

Figure A118   Pony of the Americas (POA).

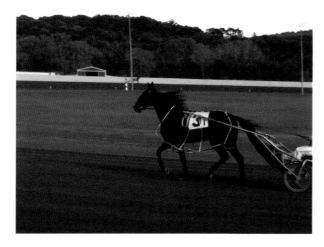

Figure A119   Standardbred. *Source*: Courtesy of Molly Brobst.

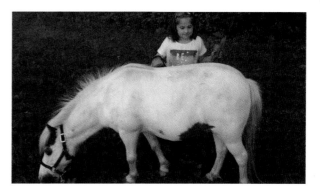

Figure A120   Shetland Pony. *Source*: Courtesy of Molly Brobst.

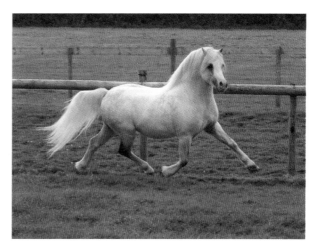

Figure A121   Welsh Pony.

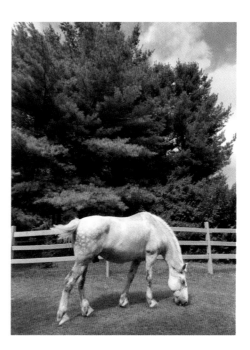

Figure A122   Percheron.

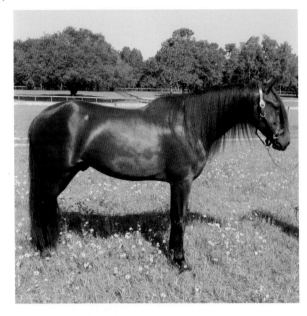

Figure A123 Cleveland Bay.

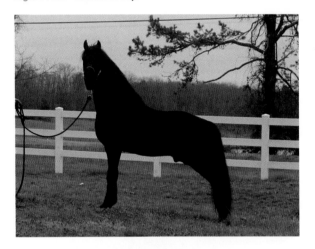

Figure A124 Tennessee Walking Horse.

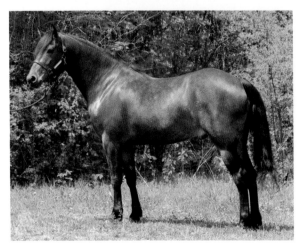

Figure A125 Morgan.

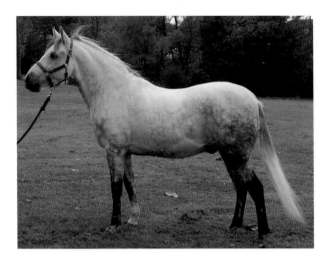

Figure A126 Paso Fino.

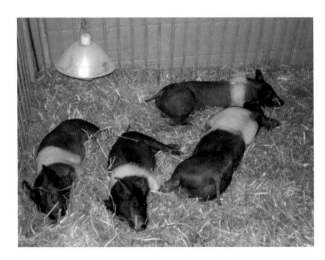

Figure A127 Hampshire.

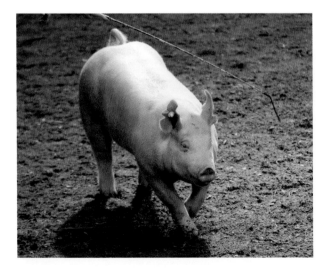

Figure A128 American Yorkshire. *Source*: Courtesy of Wendy MacDonald.

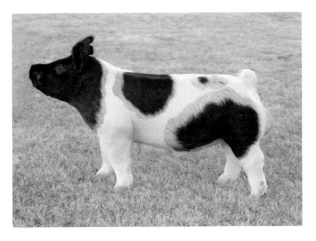

Figure A129 Spots.

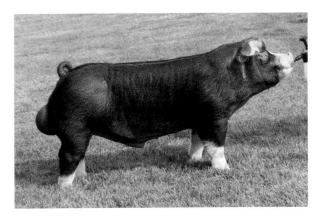

Figure A132 Berkshire.

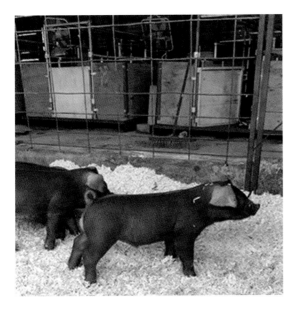

Figure A130 Duroc.

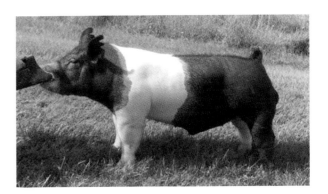

Figure A133 Saddleback.

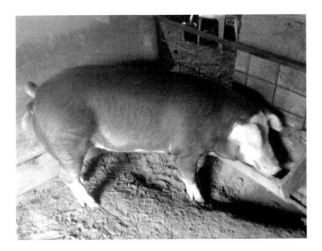

Figure A131 Hereford.

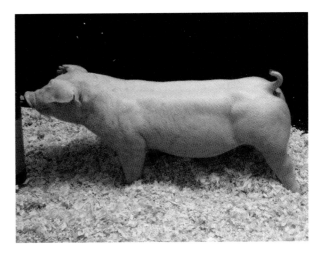

Figure A134 American Landrace.

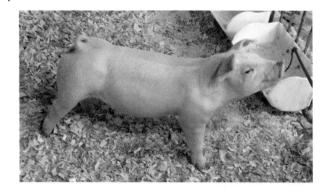

Figure A135 Chester White.

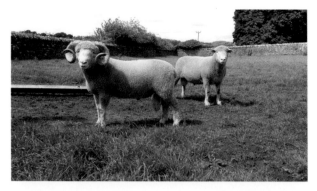

Figure A138 Rambouillet.

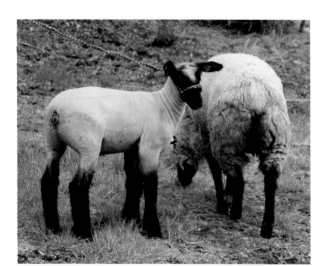

Figure A136 Suffolk. *Source*: Courtesy of Wendy MacDonald.

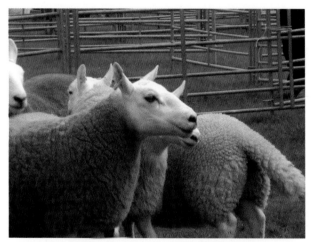

Figure A139 Cheviot.

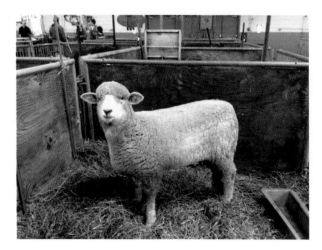

Figure A137 Corriedale.

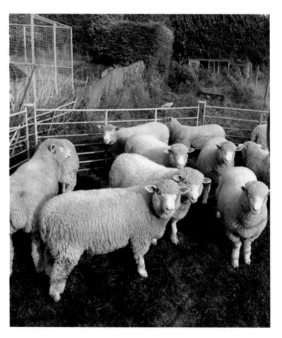

Figure A140 Dorset.

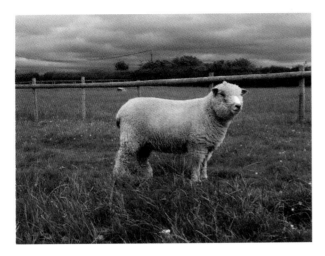

Figure A141 Southdown.

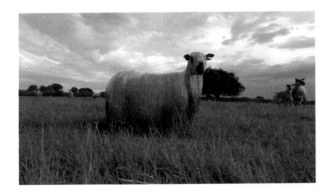

Figure A142 Lincoln.

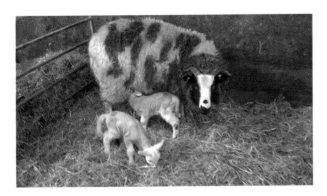

Figure A143 Jacob.

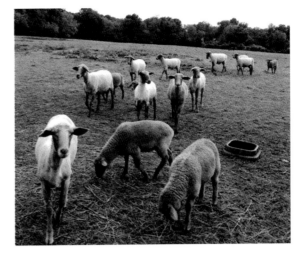

Figure A144 Tunis.

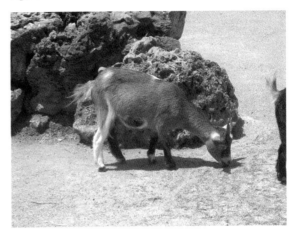

Figure A145 Pygmy.

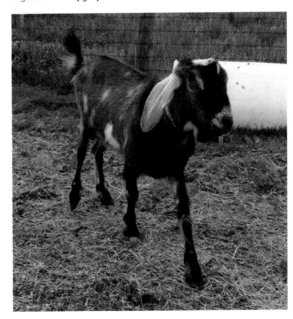

Figure A146 Nubian.

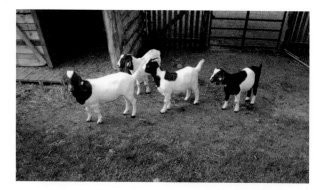

Figure A147 Boer.

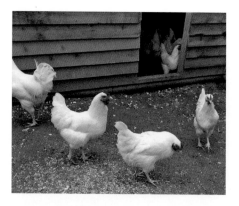

Figure A150 Leghorn.

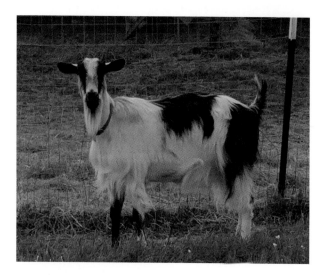

Figure A148 Alpine.

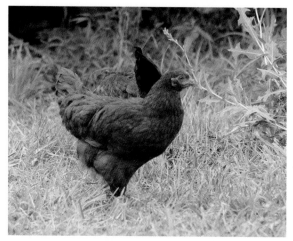

Figure A151 Rhode Island Red. *Source*: Courtesy of Wendy MacDonald.

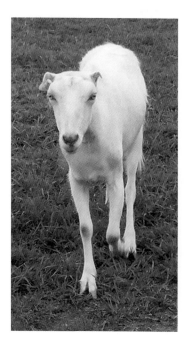

Figure A149 LaMancha.

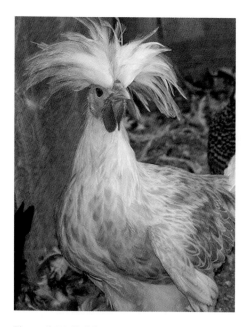

Figure A152 Polish.

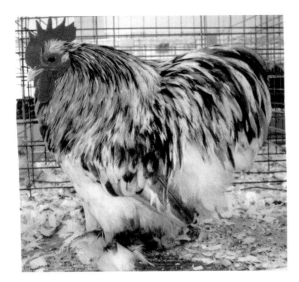

Figure A153 Cochin.

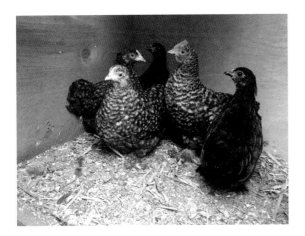

Figure A154 Bantam.

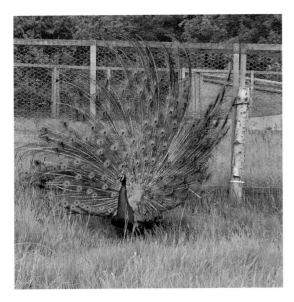

Figure A155 Peafowl/Peacock.

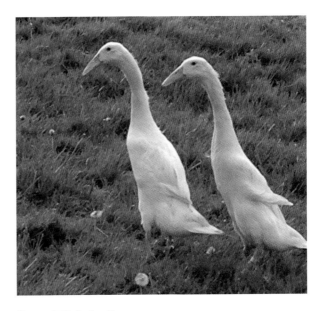

Figure A156 Indian Runner.

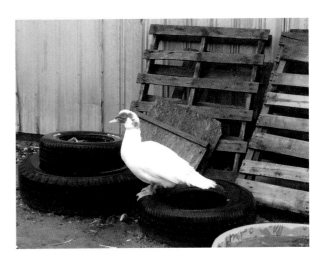

Figure A157 Muscovy. *Source*: Courtesy of Wendy MacDonald.

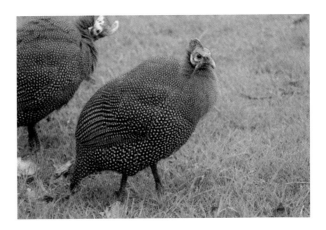

Figure A158 Guinea Fowl.

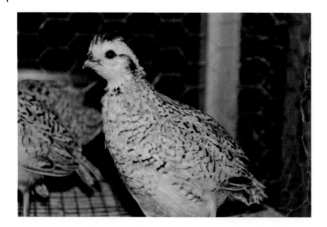

Figure A159 Quail.

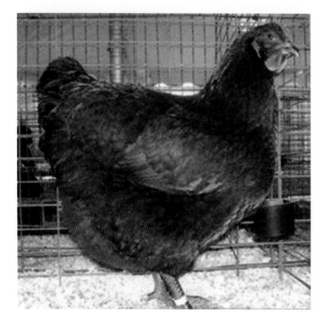

Figure A160 Jersey Giant.

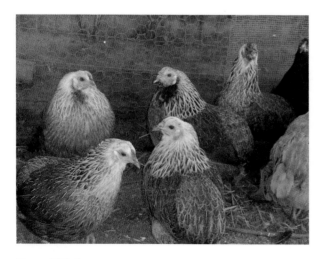

Figure A161 Araucana.

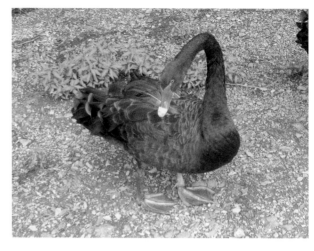

Figure A162 Swan.

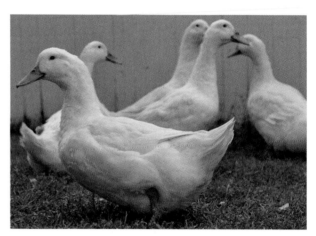

Figure A163 Pekin.

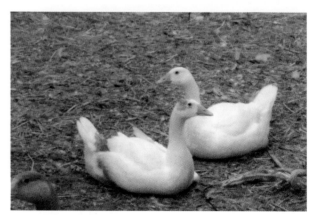

Figure A164 Embden.

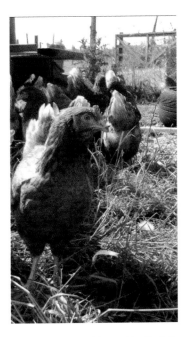

Figure A165 New Hampshire Red. *Source*: Courtesy of Wendy MacDonald.

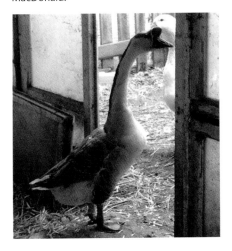

Figure A166 Chinese.

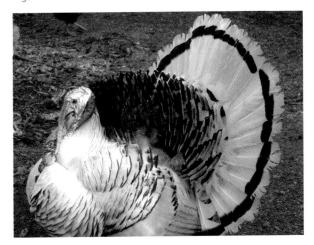

Figure A167 Royal Palm.

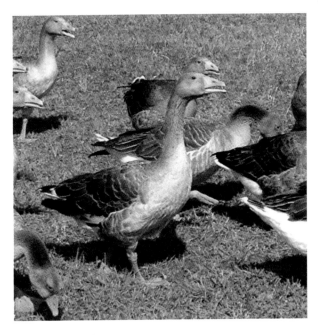

Figure A168 Toulouse.

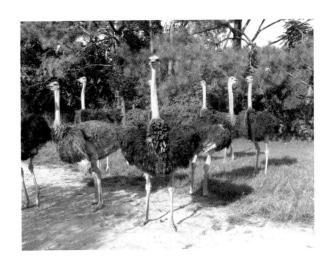

Figure A169 Ostrich.

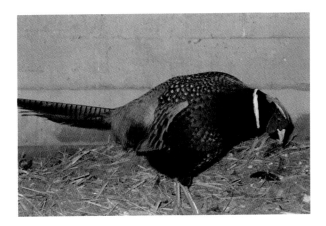

Figure A170 Pheasant.

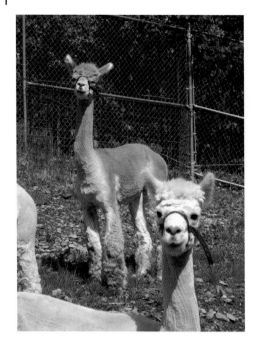

Figure A171 Alpaca.

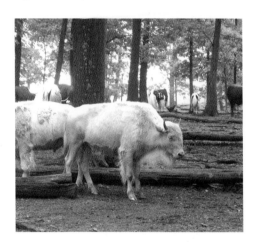

Figure A172 Beefalo.

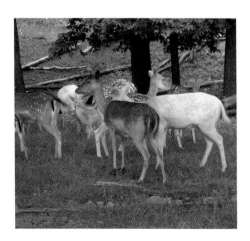

Figure A173 Fallow Deer

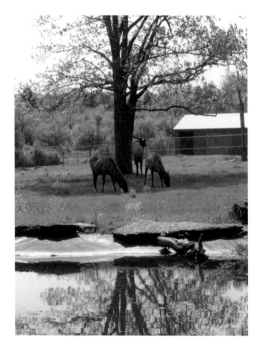

Figure A174 Elk.

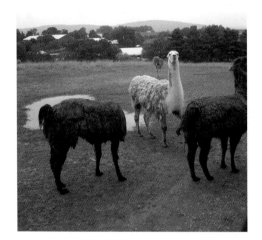

Figure A175 Llama.

Index

Abyssinian, 82
Abyssinian guinea pig, 13–14, 86
Afghan Hound, 77
African goose, 65
African Grey Parrot, 89
alligator, 27
alpaca, 71, 75, 106
Alpine, 54, 102
alternative production animal, 69
American Bullfrog, 92
American Cavy Breeders Association (ACBA), 13
American Chinchilla, 84
American Class, 58
American Curl, 83
American Dairy Goat Association (ADGA), 53
American Donkey and Mule Society, 40
American Fancy Rat and Mouse Association (AFRMA), 15
American Ferret Association (AFA), 15
American Foxhound, 79
American Goat Society (AGS), 53
American guinea pig, 13–14, 86
American Kennel Club (AKC), 1, 4
American Landrace, 42, 99
American Miniature Horse, 95
American Poultry Association (APA), 57
American Quarter Horse, 39, 95
American Rabbit Breeders Association (ARBA), 9, 13
American Reptile Association (ARA), 25
American Sable, 85
American Sheep Industry Association (ASI), 47
American Toad, 30, 93
American Yorkshire, 98
amphibian, 29–31
Ancona, 60
Andalusian, 61
Angora, 54
Angus, 34, 93
Appaloosa, 95
aquaculture, 69–70

Arabian, 96
Araucana, 60, 104
Asiatic Class, 58
Australian Shepherd, 77
avian, 21–24
Axis deer, 72
Aylesbury, 64

backfat, 41–42
bacon type, 41
ball python, 92
bantam, 60, 62–63, 103
Barbados Blackbelly, 48, 51–52
Basset Hound, 80
Bearded Dragon, 91
beefalo, 73, 106
beef cow, 33–35, 77
Belgian, 39, 96
Bengal, 82
Berkshire, 43, 99
Bernese Mountain Dog, 81
Bichon Frise, 81
bicolor, 6
bison, 69–70, 72
Black Angus, 34
Black-faced Highland, 52
Blue and Gold Macaw, 89
Bluetick Coonhound, 78
Boa Constrictor, 26, 92
Boer, 54–55, 102
Bombay, 83
Borzoi, 78
Boston Terrier, 3
Boxer, 78
Box Turtle, 27, 92
Brahma, 61
Bronze, 62, 64
Brown Swiss, 95
Buckeye, 61
Buckskin, 37
budgerigar, 89
Buff, 63
bullfrog, 30
Burmese, 84

caiman, 27
calico, 6–7
camelid, 69
Campbell, 64
Canada goose, 64–65
canary, 23, 90
Cane Corso, 81
carpet sheep breeds, 48, 52
cashmere, 54
cat, 5–8, 77
Catalana, 61
Cat Fanciers Association (CFA), 5
catfish farming, 69, 72
cattle, 33–35
championship class, 5–6
Charolais, 94
Chesapeake Bay Retriever, 80
Chester White, 42–43, 100
Cheviot, 47, 49, 100
chevon, 53
chicken, 57–58, 60–62
Chihuahua, 4
chinchilla, 18, 88
Chinchilla Breeders Organization (CBO), 15
Chinese, 105
Cleveland Bay, 98
Cochin, 60–61, 103
cockatiel, 90
cockatoo, 23
Collie, 2
Columbia, 47, 51
Continental Class, 58
Cornish, 60–61
Corn Snake, 91
Coronet guinea pig, 13
Corriedale, 47–48, 51, 100
Cotswold, 50
Crested, 63–64
crocodile, 27
cross-bred wool sheep, 47, 51
Curly Coated Retriever, 81
cylindrical, 9–11

Veterinary Guide to Animal Breeds, First Edition. Beth Vanhorn.
© 2018 John Wiley & Sons, Inc. Published 2018 by John Wiley & Sons, Inc.
Companion website: www.wiley.com/go/vanhorn/breeds

dairy cow, 33–35, 77
dairy goat, 53
Debouillet, 49
deer, 69
deer farm, 71–72
Delaware, 61
diluted, 6
Doberman Pinscher, 78
dog, 1–4, 77
donkey, 37, 39–40, 96
Dorper, 51
Dorset, 47, 49, 100
draft breed, 38–39
duck, 57–59, 63–65
Dumbo Rat, 87
Dun, 37–38
Duroc, 42, 99
Dutch, 85
Dwarf Hotot, 84

ecdysis, 25–26
Eclectus parrot, 22
Egyptian goose, 64–65
elk, 74–75, 106
Embden, 59, 65, 104
emu, 59, 65–66
English Class, 58
English Setter, 78
English Springer Spaniel, 3, 79
equine, 37–40
exotic, 83

fallow deer, 73–74, 106
ferret, 18, 77, 88
fine wool sheep, 47, 49
Finnish Landrace, 50
fleece, 49
French Bulldog, 81
frog, 29–30
full-arch, 9–11
fur sheep breeds, 48

Galloway, 93
gerbil, 17–18, 77, 88
German Shepherd Dog, 79
goat, 53–56, 77
Golden hamster, 16
goose, 57, 59, 64–66
Great Dane, 82
Greater Swiss Mountain Dog, 82
Green Anole, 92
Green Iguana, 91
Green Treefrog, 93
Green Winged Macaw, 90
Greyhound, 2
Guernsey, 95
guinea fowl, 59, 66–67, 103
guinea pig, 13–14, 77

hairless, 6–7, 87
hair sheep breeds, 47–48
Hampshire, 43–44, 47, 50, 98
hamster, 16–17, 77
ham type, 41–42
Hanoverian, 97
hare, 9–10
Havana Brown, 83
hedgehog, 18, 88
herding, 1–2
Hereford, 34, 42–43, 93, 99
Highland, 93
Himalayan, 83
Himalayan guinea pig, 13
Holland, 62
Holland Lop, 85
Holstein, 34, 94
hooded rat, 88
hoof, 37–38
horse, 37–38, 77
hound, 2
household pet class, 5
hunter horse, 39
Hyacinth Macaw, 90

Indian Runner, 64, 103
International Hedgehog Association
    (IHA), 15
Irish Wolfhound, 82

Jacob, 101
Jersey, 35
Jersey Giant, 61–62, 104
jird, 17

Karakul, 52
Katahdin, 48–49, 52
kitten class, 5–6

Labrador Retriever, 79
lagomorph, 9
LaMancha, 54–55, 102
Landrace, 44
Langshan, 62
Leghorn, 61, 102
light breed, 38
Lincoln, 51, 101
lizard, 26, 77
llama, 75, 106
longhair, 6–7
long wool sheep, 47, 50

Magpie, 64
Map Turtle, 91
Mastiff, 79
meat goat, 53
Mediterranean Class, 58
medium wool sheep, 47, 49

Merino, 47, 49
Milking Shorthorn, 95
miniature donkey, 40
miniature horse, 39
miniature mule, 40, 96
Minnesota Companion Bird Association
    (MCBA), 21
miscellaneous class, 4–5
mohair, 54
Moluccan Cockatoo, 89
Mongolian gerbil, 17
Montadale, 50
Morgan, 98
mouse, 15–16
mule, 37, 40
Muscovy, 64–65, 103

National Cattleman's Beef Association
    (NCBA), 33
National Gerbil Society (NGS), 15
National Hamster Council (NHC), 15
National Pork Producers Council
    (NPPC), 41
National Swine Registry (NSR), 41
Netherland Dwarf, 85
New Hampshire Red, 61–62, 105
newt, 31
New World birds, 22–23
non-sporting, 2–3
Norway rat, 15
Nubian, 54–55, 101

Old World birds, 22–23
ostrich, 59, 65–66, 105
Oxford, 47, 50

pack animal, 75
Paint, 38, 96
Palomino, 37–38
parakeet, 89
Parson Russel Terrier, 3
parti-color, 6
Paso Fino, 98
Passerine, 23
peach faced lovebird, 91
peafowl, 59, 66–67, 103
Pekin, 59, 64, 104
Pembroke Welsh Corgi, 78
Percheron, 97
Persian, 83
Peruvian guinea pig, 13–14, 87
pheasant, 105
Pietrain, 44
pigeon, 59, 66–67
Pilgrim, 64–65
Pinto, 38
Plymouth Rock, 59, 61–62
Poland China, 43

Polish, 61–62, 85, 102
Pomeranian, 79
pony, 38
Pony of Americas (POA), 39, 97
premiership class, 5
Psittacine, 23
Purebred Dairy Cattle Association (PDCA), 33
Pygmy, 55, 101
python, 26

quail, 59–60, 67, 104

rabbit, 9–11, 77
Rambouillet, 47–49, 100
rat, 15–16
ratite, 21, 23, 59, 65
Rat and Mouse Club of America (AMCA), 15
Red Angus, 93
Redbone Coonhound, 80
Redcap, 63red deer, 74
Red Eared Slider, 91
red-spotted newt, 31
reptile, 25–27
Rex, 85
Rex guinea pig, 13
rhea, 59, 65, 67
Rhode Island Red, 61–62, 102
Rhodesian Ridgeback, 80
Roan, 38
Romney, 51
Rottweiler, 4
Royal Palm, 64, 105
ruminant, 33, 47, 53
Russian Blue, 84
Russian Dwarf, 87

Saanen, 55–56
Saddleback, 99
Saint Bernard, 82
salamander, 30
Salmonella, 25, 29

salmon farming, 72
Saluki, 80
Satin, 86
scutes, 25
semi-arch, 9–11
Senegal Parrot, 89
sheep, 47–52
Shetland Pony, 97
shorthair, 6–7
Shorthorn, 94
Siamese, 84
Siberian Husky, 80
sika deer, 74
Silkie guinea pig, 13
Simmental, 94
skinny guinea pig, 14, 86
Slate, 63–64
small commercial, 9–11
snake, 26, 77
Society for the Study of Reptiles and Amphibians (SSAR), 25, 29
Southdown, 47, 50, 101
sporting, 2–3
spots, 43, 99
spotted salamander, 30
Standardbred, 97
standard commercial, 9–11
Standard of Perfection, 57, 60, 62
Standard Poodle, 81
St. Croix, 48, 52
stock breed, 38
Suffolk, 47–48, 50, 100
Sultan, 63
Sun Conure, 90
Sussex, 63
swan, 104
Swedish, 64
swine, 41–45
Syrian hamster, 16

tabby, 6–7
Tamworth, 43–44

Tan, 86
Targhee, 51
Teddy Bear Hamster, 88
Teddy guinea pig, 14, 87
Tennessee Walking Horse, 98
terrier, 2–3
Texas Longhorn, 94
Texel guinea pig, 14, 87
Thoroughbred, 96
toad, 29–30
Toggenburg, 56
tortoiseshell, 6–7
Toulouse, 65, 105
toy, 2–3
trout farming, 72–73
Tunis, 50–51, 101
turkey, 57–58, 62–64
Turkish Angora, 84
turtle, 27, 77

United States Department of Agriculture (USDA), 33

veiled chameleon, 92
venison, 69, 74
veteran class, 5–6

warmblood, 38
waterfowl, 57
Welsh Pony, 97
White Chinese, 65–66
White Crested guinea pig, 14, 86
White Holland, 63–64
White-Tailed deer, 74
Winter White Hamster, 89
working, 2, 4
Wyandotte, 62–63

Yellow Head Amazon, 23
Yorkshire, 44

Zebra Finch, 90